MEDICAL
INTELLIGENCE
UNIT

CONDUITS FOR MYOCARDIAL REVASCULARIZATION

Michel Carrier, MD, FRCSC

L. Conrad Pelletier, MD, FRCSC, FACS

University of Montreal

R.G. LANDES COMPANY
AUSTIN

Medical Intelligence Unit

CONDUITS FOR MYOCARDIAL REVASCULARIZATION

R.G. LANDES COMPANY
Austin / Georgetown

CRC Press is the exclusive worldwide distributor of publications of the Medical Intelligence Unit.
CRC Press, 2000 Corporate Blvd. NW, Boca Raton, FL 33431. Phone: 407/994-0555.

Submitted: March 1993
Published: April 1993

Production: Carol Harwell
Copy Editor: Constance Kerkaporta

Please address all inquiries to the Publisher:
R.G. Landes Company
909 Pine Street
Georgetown, TX 78626
or
P.O. Box 4858
Austin, TX 78765
Phone: 512/ 863 7762
FAX: 512/ 863 0081

ISBN 1-879702-66-5
CATALOG # LN-0266

CONTRIBUTORS

Martial G. Bourassa, MD, FRCSC
Professor of Medicine
University of Montreal
Senior Cardiologist and Director of Medical Affairs
Montreal Heart Institute
Montreal, Quebec, Canada

Michel Carrier, MD, FRCSC
Assistant Professor of Surgery
Scholar of the FRSQ
University of Montreal
Surgeon, Montreal Heart Institute
Montreal, Quebec, Canada

Raymond Cartier, MD, FRCSC
Assistant Professor of Surgery
University of Montreal
Surgeon, Montreal Heart Institute
Montreal, Quebec, Canada

L. Conrad Pelletier, MD, FRCSC, FACS
Professor of Surgery and Chairman of the Department of Surgery
University of Montreal
Surgeon, Montreal Heart Institute
Montreal, Quebec, Canada

Louis Perrault, MD, FRCSC
Senior Resident in Cardiovascular and Thoracic Surgery
University of Montreal
Montreal Heart Institute
Montreal, Quebec, Canada

PREFACE

Coronary artery bypass grafting has had a major impact on the management of patients with severe coronary artery disease during the last 25 years. Early in its development bypass surgery became established as an effective and relatively safe method of restoring myocardial perfusion and relieving myocardial ischemia and angina pectoris. The large clinical trials completed during the 1980s demonstrated clearly that bypass surgery is capable of improving long-term survival in selected patient subsets. The frequency of coronary artery bypass grafting increased rapidly during the first 15 years of its existence and has continued to expand during the last 10 years albeit at a more reduced pace. Currently, coronary artery bypass grafting is by far the most frequently performed cardiac surgical procedure.

However, the technique of coronary artery bypass grafting has undergone major changes over the years. First, the patient population undergoing the procedure has evolved and expanded. Compared to the early years of bypass surgery, advanced age, female gender, diabetes mellitus, triple-vessel disease, left main coronary stenosis and abnormal left ventricular function are common features of patients currently undergoing bypass surgery. As a result a much higher risk population is operated upon now than previously. In addition, because of the palliative nature of revascularization procedures a significant proportion of patients currently undergoing bypass surgery has had prior coronary artery bypass grafting or prior coronary angioplasty. In addition to significantly increasing the risk of bypass surgery, these reinterventions pose many technical problems, one of which may be the lack of availability of bypass conduits and the need to resort to the new types of grafts.

The operative technique has also evolved and, overall, has become safer for the high-risk patients now undergoing the operation. One of the main factors which can be readily identified is effective myocardial protection through the use of cardioplegia.

Finally, as discussed in detail throughout this monograph, the choice of bypass conduits has undergone a major evolution during the last 10 to 15 years. Although saphenous vein grafts were routinely used during the early years of bypass surgery because of their ready availability and ease of surgical removal, we learned in the 1970s and early 1980s that they often have a limited longevity because of the development of thrombosis, hyperplasia and atherosclerosis. In contrast, internal mammary artery grafts rarely develop atherosclerosis and they have much higher long-term patency rates than saphenous vein grafts. Patients with a single internal mammary artery graft to the left anterior descending artery have a significantly better long-term survival than those with only saphenous vein grafts. Patients with bilateral internal mammary artery grafts have less coronary events than those with a single internal mammary artery graft. These observations have led to changes in practice patterns which began in the early 1980s and have progressed until now. Currently at our institution, more than 90% of patients undergoing coronary artery bypass grafting receive at least one internal mammary artery graft to the left anterior descending artery and 45% receive bilateral internal mammary artery grafts.

During the last five or six years new types of arterial grafts such as the right gastroepiploic artery and the inferior epigastric artery grafts have been introduced and used for multiple arterial bypass grafting. These conduits are particularly useful in younger patients with severe hypercholesterolemia or diabetes mellitus in whom atherosclerosis is more likely to develop and to produce occlusion of saphenous vein grafts and in patients undergoing reoperation or in those in whom the availability of other conduits is limited. Although early results are encouraging, the long-term angiographic patency rates of these grafts have not yet been reported.

Despite the more widespread use of arterial grafts there are good reasons to believe that saphenous vein grafts will remain in constant demand. These reasons include the more difficult technique of arterial bypass grafting and the increasing number of bypass procedures in elderly patients, in patients with unstable angina and in those requiring multiple bypass grafts. Therefore strategies for improving the late patency of saphenous vein grafts remain of critical importance. Routine postoperative use of antiplatelet drugs results in improved early vein graft patency. There is also evidence suggesting that lowering blood lipids after bypass surgery may reduce late vein graft failure. This avenue is being investigated in at least one large prospective randomized trial.

Coronary artery bypass grafting is one of the two currently accepted alternative methods of myocardial revascularization in patients with coronary artery disease. Percutaneous transluminal coronary angioplasty was introduced approximately 15 years ago and has gained widespread acceptance as a less invasive method of myocardial revascularization in a large number of selected patients with coronary artery disease. Currently, coronary angioplasty is performed slightly more frequently than bypass surgery, although the majority of the candidates are still patients with single-vessel coronary artery disease. Complete or optimal revascularization in patients with multivessel disease is achieved much more frequently following coronary artery bypass grafting than following coronary angioplasty. Nevertheless, balloon angioplasty has been shown to be effective in relieving angina pectoris and to be probably as safe as bypass surgery in selected patients with multivessel disease. In contrast to bypass surgery, however, its long-term results have not been evaluated in prospective randomized studies.

During the last few years balloon angioplasty has been assisted or supplemented by several new devices which include catheter atherectomy, coronary stents and excimer laser angioplasty. These new techniques may be more effective than balloon angioplasty in the treatment of complex coronary stenoses. Their short-term results are often encouraging. However, their long-term efficacy is totally unknown.

One of the major challenges of the future in patients with multivessel disease requiring myocardial revascularization will be to carefully assess the long-term effects on mortality, morbidity and the degree of revascularization of balloon angioplasty assisted by new devices versus coronary artery bypass grafting using one of the several arterial grafts. Such comparisons are already ongoing and new large randomized clinical trials will be needed in the future.

Martial G. Bourassa

CONTENTS

INTRODUCTION

Michel Carrier
L. Conrad Pelletier

Coronary artery bypass grafting has become one of the most commonly performed surgical procedures in North America. The high prevalence of coronary artery disease and its dramatic personal and social impact, particularly in the middle-aged patient, together with the several major improvements in surgical techniques throughout the last 25 years, have paved the way to the rapid development and progress of coronary artery surgery. Nowadays, despite the availability of better medical therapy and of coronary angioplasty, surgical revascularization of the myocardium remains the treatment of choice for the most advanced forms of coronary artery disease and for the most severely disabled patients. Because of the very large case load that will likely continue to be generated for this surgical procedure in years ahead, the rapidly growing cost to the health care system is becoming a major concern for health care planners, governments and third-party payers. Long-term efficacy of coronary artery bypass grafting will therefore be a key issue that will be scrutinized by those involved in the allocation of scarce resources.

The choice of conduits for myocardial revascularization has been shown to be one of the main determinant factors of the long-term results of surgical treatment. The saphenous veins, the internal mammary arteries, the right gastroepiploic and the inferior epigastric arteries, as well as a number of other conduits have been used to bypass coronary artery lesions over the years. The objective of this monograph is to review the clinical and angiographic results obtained with these various conduits and to discuss the respective role they are likely to play in coronary artery bypass grafting today.

Our comments and opinions are based on the extensive clinical experience developed throughout the last 25 years at the Montreal Heart Institute, as well as on that of several other centers that have participated in the progress of coronary artery surgery. The determinant influence of the large multicenter trials on the evolution of numerous basic concepts regarding the surgical approach to coronary artery disease must also be stressed and will be largely discussed.

Numerous researchers from our institution have been closely involved in the development and the evaluation of coronary artery bypass grafting since the very early days, and we are indebted to these pioneers for their dedication and enthusiasm in procuring optimal quality care for the coronary patient and for their significant contribution at solving the many clinical issues throughout all those years. We wish to commend these colleagues for their leadership and accomplishment.

CHAPTER 2

THE SAPHENOUS VEIN GRAFT: WHAT HAVE WE LEARNED FROM THE PAST 25 YEARS?

L. Conrad Pelletier

HISTORY

In medicine, the ultimate achievement of applying new knowledge to the treatment of patients rests at the end of a long road of tedious and tenacious work in research laboratories, and myocardial revascularization has been no exception to that rule (Table 1). From Alexis Carrel[1] who developed the technical principles of vascular anastomoses and achieved the first direct anastomosis of an artery to the left coronary artery in 1910, achievements for which he was awarded the Nobel Prize for Medicine in 1912, to clinical application in coronary artery grafting, over 50 years had elapsed. The idea of improving coronary blood flow through surgical means was almost forgotten until an American surgeon from Cleveland, Claude Beck,[2] published a paper on the "production of a collateral circulation to the heart" in 1935. He observed that abrasion of the epicardium and dusting with an irritating powder stimulated the development of collateral vessels to the myocardium from the pectoralis muscle used as a pedicled graft to wrap the heart.

Some 15 years later, in 1950, Arthur Vineberg,[3] a Canadian surgeon from Montreal, reported a technique he had developed experimentally to implant the internal mammary artery directly into the myocardium in order to stimulate the development of new anastomoses with the myocardial venous sinusoids. During the same period, the idea of directly anastomosing a blood vessel to coronary arteries was again explored, and another Canadian surgeon, Gordon Murray[4] from Toronto, was the first to report successful anastomosis of an arterial graft to a coronary artery in dogs in 1954. A direct anastomosis of the internal mammary artery to the circumflex coronary artery with long-term survival was achieved in the dog by Alan Thal in 1956.[5] Until then, the feasibility of anastomosing bypass grafts directly to the coronary arteries had been demonstrated, but the procedure had remained in the laboratory and had not yet crossed the bridge to human application. A major piece of information was still lacking before the technique could be applied to the treatment of coronary artery disease in man: knowledge of precise anatomical distribution of coronary lesions.

Table 1. Major Landmarks in the Development of Coronary Artery Bypass Grafting

Experimental

1910 - A. Carrel	-	vascular anastomoses
1935 - C. Beck	-	production of collateral vessels
1950 - A. Vineberg	-	mammary artery implant in myocardium
1954 - G. Murray	-	direct anastomosis to coronary artery
1956 - A. Thal	-	mammary to coronary artery anastomosis

Clinical

1958 - M. Sones	-	selective coronary angiography
1961 - A. Senning	-	coronary artery endarterectomy
1962 - A. Vineberg	-	the "Vineberg operation" in man
1964 - H. Garrett	-	first vein graft to coronary artery
1966 - V. Kolessov	-	first mammary to coronary anastomosis
1967 - R. Favaloro	-	saphenous vein graft for coronary bypass
1968 - G. Green	-	first mammary to coronary anastomosis in USA

This new step forward was to occur at the Cleveland Clinic, toward the end of 1958 when Mason Sones,[6] by mere luck while attempting to do a supravalvular aortography, actually performed the first ever selective coronary angiography. This was to be a major landmark in the subsequent development of surgical treatment of coronary artery disease. Initially, coronary angiography proved that Vineberg was right, and that the internal mammary artery implanted in the myocardium (the Vineberg operation) remained patent and that anastomoses with the venous sinusoids of the myocardium did, in fact, develop. However, whether this operation could actually relieve myocardial ischemia or not was still an open question, but since no other treatment was available the Vineberg procedure was widely used between

1962 and 1968. Simultaneously, other approaches were being sought. In 1961, Senning[7] reported a case of coronary endarterectomy with vein patch enlargement of the coronary artery, the success of which was demonstrated at coronary angiography. The technique of patch graft enlargement of coronary arteries was further refined by Donald Effler at the Cleveland Clinic.[8]

The modern era of coronary artery bypass grafting was opened by Garrett in 1964 when he performed in Houston the first saphenous vein graft to a coronary artery after being unable to do a coronary artery endarterectomy in his patient. It was nine years before this unique experience was reported.[9] In the meantime this approach had been more or less forgotten until the Cleveland Clinic surgical team with René Favaloro and Donald Effler[10] performed in 1967 their first of a large series of coronary artery bypass grafting with saphenous vein grafts, and popularized its use. In Milwaukee, Dudley Johnson[11] rapidly became one of the major supporters of the technique, proposing an aggressive attitude in the surgical treatment of multivessel coronary disease, an experience that was published in 1970. In Canada, the first patient to undergo coronary artery bypass with a saphenous vein graft was operated upon in September 1969 by Pierre Grondin, at the Montreal Heart Institute.[12]

Whereas a consensus had rapidly developed among surgeons regarding the value of bypassing diseased coronary arteries, opinions differed as to what was the most proper conduit to use. Professor Vasilii Kolessov, then working in Leningrad (which has now recovered its former name of St. Petersburg), published in 1967 in the *Journal of Cardiovascular and Thoracic Surgery* a paper entitled "Mammary artery-coronary artery anastomosis as a method of treatment for angina pectoris".[13] The Russian pioneer had performed the operation for the first time in 1966, and was reporting on six cases with five survivors. This was the first report ever of direct anastomosis of the internal mammary artery to a coronary artery in man. Coronary angiography was not available to Kolessov who had to rely solely on clinical, electrocardiographic and operative evaluation, and the operation was performed without the use of cardiopulmonary bypass.

In 1968, George Green[14] in New York described the modern technique of internal mammary artery to coronary artery bypass grafting and reported the first clinical cases in North America. His major contribution has been to be the first one to recognize, as early as 1970, the superiority of mammary arterial grafts over vein grafts for coronary bypass and to have strongly and tenaciously recommended its use in preference to saphenous vein grafts ever since.[15] It was not long before Floyd Loop at the Cleveland Clinic[16] also agreed to the value of the internal mammary artery and starting in 1971 used this conduit on a regular basis. In his report on the initial series of 25 cases, he stressed several advantages of the internal mammary graft, namely that this artery was free from atherosclerotic disease, that it had a diameter similar to that of coronary arteries, and that an artery-to-artery anastomosis probably had a better longevity than a veno-arterial anastomosis.

While the value of coronary artery bypass grafting has been rapidly accepted by cardiac surgeons, cardiologists have been much more reluctant to recognize its place in the treatment of coronary artery disease. Never has a surgical procedure of any kind been submitted to such scrutiny, to so numerous studies, to such close monitoring and surveillance as has been the case for coronary artery bypass grafting. Whereas in the beginning this operation had been the subject of much criticism and reluctance outside of the surgical community, it finally became widely accepted as a valuable and scientifically sound treatment of coronary artery disease in the mid-70s. Since then, direct myocardial revascularization has been the fastest growing surgical procedure in North America. It is now performed at a rate of approximately 160 per 100,000 population in the United States, and 70 per 100,000 population inCamada (personal communication). The indications for the operation have been better defined, and the clinical and angiographic outcomes have been the object of incalculable studies and reports. After 25 years, there is an overwhelming amount of data indicating that coronary artery bypass grafting has been among the most useful and rewarding treatments, albeit palliative, of coronary artery disease, when properly applied and performed. It might even be one of the factors responsible for the recent decrease in the mortality from this disease in North America.

CLINICAL RESULTS OF CORONARY ARTERY BYPASS GRAFTING

Because of the huge experience accumulated worldwide with the use of saphenous vein grafts in myocardial revascularization, the results with this type of conduit have become the standard against which other conduits have to be compared. The data discussed in this chapter will therefore mainly concern results obtained with saphenous vein grafts.

Results of surgical treatment of coronary artery disease have been evaluated in terms of survival, risk of myocardial infarction, recovery of myocardial function, quality of life, and return to productive activities in the society. It was initially hoped that coronary bypass surgery could improve all of these variables, but convincing evidence appeared only when the results of broad clinical studies became available in the early 1980s. Three prospective, randomized, multicenter trials have been performed between 1972 and 1980 to compare the efficacy of medical versus surgical treatment of coronary artery disease: the Veterans Administration Cooperative Study Group (VA Study) which enrolled 686 patients from 1972 to 1974,[17] the European Coronary Surgery Study Group (European Study) with an enrollment of 768 patients from 1973 to 1976,[18] and the Coronary Artery Surgery Study (CASS) with 780 patients enrolled from 1975 to 1979.[19] A total of 2234 patients were therefore randomized and followed for up to 11 to 12 years after study entry. Although all three trials had the same goal, there were some significant differences in their respective study populations that must be taken into consideration to understand the differences in their results.[20] In the VA Study there were no women and older patients were recruited. In CASS, there were no severely disabled patients, whereas some asymptomatic postmyocardial infarction patients were included. Severe stenosis of the left main coronary artery was excluded in CASS, whereas the European Study did not include patients with significant left ventricular dysfunction (ejection fraction less than 50%).

OPERATIVE RISK

In the early experience, the surgical mortality of myocardial revascularization varied from 1 to 12%, these wide differences being mainly due to

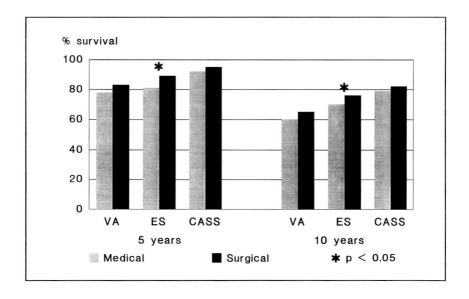

Figure 1. Overall cumulative survival of all patients 5 and 10 years after study entry in the three multicenter randomized trials. Data calculated and summarized from Varnauskas E et al,[28] Alderman EL et al,[29] and Veterans Administration Coronary Artery Bypass Surgery Cooperative Study Group.[30] VA: Veterans Administration Cooperative Study Group; ES: European Coronary Study Group; CASS: Coronary Artery Surgery Study. Only the ES trial showed a significant difference in overall survival between medical and surgical groups (p < 0.05).

patient selection.[21] Surgical morbidity was particularly related to the occurrence of perioperative myocardial infarction, with a markedly variable incidence in the literature, from 5 to as high as 23%.[22] Obviously, the different diagnostic criteria of perioperative myocardial infarction used in the various studies accounted for much of the variation in the reported incidence. However, with increasing experience, improvement in myocardial protection during operation, and better patient selection, both surgical mortality and perioperative myocardial infarction rates decreased to around 1 to 2% each, after 1980.[23,24]

SURVIVAL

Among the three studies, only the European Study[25] reported an overall better long-term survival following surgical treatment compared to medical treatment (Figure 1). When the results were broken down by the extent of coronary involvement and left ventricular impairment, patterns of survival became more consistent. Up to 12 years of follow-up, there was no significant improvement in survival with surgical treatment over that obtained with medical treatment among patients with single- and double-vessel disease in

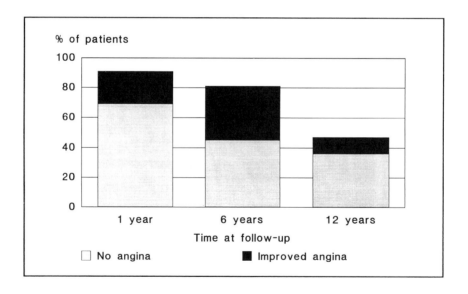

Figure 2. Changes in the degree of clinical improvement in angina with time following surgical treatment in 75 to 82 unselected patients from the Montreal Heart Institute series who underwent periodic clinical and angiographic evaluations up to 12 years. Data from Campeau L et al.[31,32]

any of the studies. In patients with triple-vessel disease, only the European study showed a significant improvement in survival with surgery compared to medical treatment. However, the difference between the two treatments became more obvious with impairment of the left ventricle. Both the VA Study and CASS found a significantly better survival at five and seven years following surgery in this subset of patients. In the CASS trial, the difference was particularly marked among patients with severe class III and IV angina pectoris, triple-vessel disease, and with an ejection fraction less than 50%. Survivals of 82% for surgical patients versus 52% for the medical treatment group after five years were reported.[26] The six-year survival of patients with an ejection fraction of less than 36% at randomization was 64% with surgery and 46% with medical treatment.[27] On the other hand, the European Study found an improvement in survival with surgery in subsets of patients with double- or triple-vessel disease and significant proximal left anterior descending artery stenosis.[28] Therefore higher risk patients appeared to benefit most from surgical revascularization in regard to late survival. This advantage of surgery in the latter group was maintained up to 10 years.[29] On the contrary, the overall survival benefit found in the European Study[28] and in the VA Study[30] tended to diminish progressively beyond five to seven years.

QUALITY OF LIFE

The relief of anginal pain has uniformly been the most rewarding achievement of surgical therapy (Figure 2). Angina improves in 90% of the patients during the first postoperative year, with approximately 70% remaining angina-free after one year.[31] However, this degree of improvement tends to decrease progressively with time. At six years, 80% are still improved, but only 45% remain asymptomatic.[31] After 12 years, this decreases further to just under 50% of improved patients, with only 35% who remain angina-free.[32] Comparative results between medical and surgical treatment in the CASS trial have shown a substantially greater proportion of surgical patients free of anginal pain, at one, three, and five years.[33] The more favorable outcome with surgical treatment was observed in all subgroups with single-, double- and triple-vessel disease. At one year, 66% of the surgical group was pain-free compared to 30% in the medical group.[34] After five years, the respective proportions were 63 and 38%. This study also indicated a greater improvement in subjective and objective functional status and lesser drug requirement following surgical treatment. However, by 10 years, the advantage of surgery becomes much less apparent, with 47% of the surgical patients remaining free of angina compared to 42% in the medical group.[34]

RETURN TO WORK

Despite the significant improvement in exercise tolerance following surgical treatment, data from CASS[34] and from the European Study[35] failed to demonstrate a better work status with surgery. In a group of working-age males, only two-thirds eventually returned to work following surgery, the peak proportion being reached after two years.[36] Several socioeconomic factors were identified as having a strong negative impact on the postoperative work status, namely a long preoperative period of unemployment, an occupation requiring strenuous physical efforts and a low level of education. Clinical variables of significance included associated noncardiovascular diseases, severity of angina and total duration of the disease preoperatively. However, under favorable circumstances, that is in patients with a short preoperative period of inactivity and with higher education and income, more than 75% are back to work at one year.[37] Therefore, individualized postoperative rehabilitation programs directed toward patients with a poor prognosis for return to work may help to improve this outcome.

MYOCARDIAL INFARCTION

Although it was initially hoped that surgical revascularization of the myocardium might decrease the incidence of myocardial infarction, no study has succeeded to demonstrate that this goal had been achieved postoperatively. On the contrary, all three randomized trials have found a very similar cumulative incidence of myocardial infarction of 14 to 15% after five years following operation compared to between 11 and 14% in the medical group.[34,35,38] Therefore, there is no evidence yet that surgery does prevent myocardial infarction, although the lack of difference between medically and surgically treated patients may be due at least in part to the incidence of perioperative myocardial infarction.

IMPROVEMENT IN MYOCARDIAL FUNCTION

A large number of studies have analyzed the changes in myocardial function postoperatively with conflicting results. Left ventricular function has been evaluated either by the regional wall motion technique or by global ejection fraction analysis. Improvement in left ventricular wall motion after surgical treatment has been reported in 10 to 65% of the patients, and worsening has been found in 3 to 40%.[39] Mean resting global left ventricular ejection fraction does not improve following surgical treatment, although individual patients may show an increase or a decrease in ejection fraction. However, in these studies, the average ejection fraction was also normal preoperatively. On the contrary, most studies found a significant improvement in exercise ejection fraction following surgery, by 6 to 16%, indicating that exercise-induced ischemia was effectively alleviated by surgical treatment.[39]

SPECIAL SITUATIONS

Left Main Coronary Artery Disease

This is the group of patients in whom the benefit of surgery in terms of survival is most striking. At seven years, a 77% survival among patients with a stenosis of 50% or more of the left main artery who underwent surgical treatment, compared to a survival of 48% in the medical group, was reported as early as 1978.[40] The difference was even more striking when only patients treated after 1972 were taken into account (90% versus 50% survival in favor of the surgical group). This was corroborated by the VA Study which showed that the difference was greatest in high-risk patients, with a 3.5-year survival of 88% with surgery versus 44% with medical treatment.[41]

Unstable Angina

It is now generally recognized that emergent surgery is rarely necessary in patients with unstable angina. In 1978, the Cleveland Clinic group[42] reported on a series of 100 consecutive patients who underwent emergency revascularization for unstable angina. The operative mortality was 4% and the rate of perioperative myocardial infarction was 18%. The authors concluded with a word of caution suggesting that a longer period of stabilization preoperatively may decrease the risk of infarction at or after surgery and that a decline in morbidity could be expected with elective rather than emergent surgery in these patients. These results were very similar to those of other randomized studies comparing medical and surgical treatment.[43] Better medical treatment, particularly the systematic use of aspirin, heparin, intravenous nitroglycerin, and mechanical support with intra-aortic balloon pumping have made it possible to control most patients presenting with unstable angina.[44] When satisfactory control of angina is obtained with medical treatment and/or mechanical support, surgery can be safely postponed, thus permitting the patients to undergo surgery in a nonischemic state. Otherwise, urgent surgery may be required. Long-term results after surgical treatment are similar to those obtained in chronic stable angina, with an improved survival in patients with triple-vessel disease and in those with left ventricular dysfunction.[45]

Myocardial Infarction

Emergent coronary artery bypass grafting has been recommended by some in the treatment of acute evolving myocardial infarction.[46] However, at the present time, there is no evidence that surgery has a role in the treatment of uncomplicated hemodynamically stable acute myocardial infarction, and therefore this approach remains experimental.

On the other hand, patients with persistent ischemia after myocardial infarction represent a particularly high-risk group. Limited treadmill stress testing after acute myocardial infarction has been shown to have a significant prognostic value.[47] One-year mortality rates of 2% in patients with a negative test and of 27% with a positive test have been found, with sudden death being 25 times more frequent in the latter group. Persistent anginal pain or a positive limited stress test are indications of postinfarction residual ischemia and are currently considered indications for immediate surgical treatment. Very good early results have been reported, particularly when the operation can be postponed until after the first week following infarction, and late results are comparable to those of patients with stable angina.[48]

Asymptomatic Patients

In a retrospective study, little benefit was found in 55 patients who underwent prophylactic coronary surgery and were followed for four to eight years.[49] This was confirmed by a CASS report indicating that in patients with mild angina and in those who remain asymptomatic after myocardial infarction, surgical treatment does not prolong life nor prevent myocardial infarction, compared to medical therapy.[50] Most patients with asymptomatic coronary artery disease or with few symptoms are therefore not candidates for surgical revascularization. Exceptions to that rule are patients with significant left main coronary artery stenosis, patients with severe proximal triple-vessel disease and left ventricular dysfunction, and those with a postmyocardial infarction positive stress test. The optimal management of patients with silent significant myocardial ischemia is not yet firmly established. However, it is generally agreed at this time that, when silent ischemia is clearly induced, the patient should undergo coronary angiography and surgery be considered according to coronary lesions.

Elderly Patients

This is a growing population group and the demand for coronary artery bypass grafting in older patients has increased steadily throughout the last decade. In this group, surgical mortality and morbidity from noncardiac complications are substantially more common than in the younger population group, thus stressing the need for careful patient selection.[51] The long-term results in regard to improvement of angina and quality of life are excellent and compare to the results obtained with younger patients.[52]

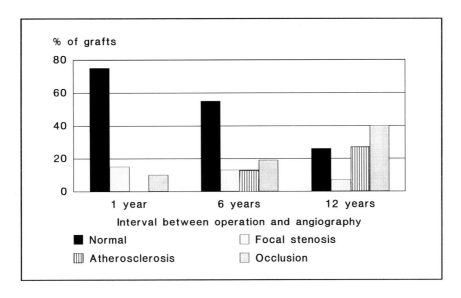

Figure 3. Changes in saphenous vein grafts at sequential angiographic examinations of 109 grafts in 60 patients of the Montreal Heart Institute cohort. Data from Campeau L et al.[55]

LATE ANGIOGRAPHIC ASSESSMENT OF SAPHENOUS VEIN GRAFTS AND OF PROGRESSION OF CORONARY ARTERY DISEASE

The progressive loss of improvement of angina that occurs one to seven years after coronary bypass surgery with saphenous vein grafts has been correlated with graft deterioration and progression of atherosclerotic coronary artery disease.[31] Over the past 20 years, a large number of studies have evaluated the long-term fate of saphenous vein grafts and found that the degree of clinical improvement was inversely correlated to late graft occlusion and disease.

PATENCY OF SAPHENOUS VEIN GRAFT

Data from the CASS randomized trial indicate a 90% patency of grafts within two months of surgery.[53] All grafts were patent in 81% of the patients, and 97% had at least one patent graft. At 18 months, the graft patency rate was 82%, and it remained the same at 60 months.

Among the first 600 patients who underwent coronary artery bypass grafting between 1969 and 1973 at the Montreal Heart Institute, 400 had angiographic evaluation of the bypass grafts less than one month after surgery, 237 were restudied after one year, and 69 had another angiographic evaluation after three years.[54] The cumulative patency rate was 87% at one month,

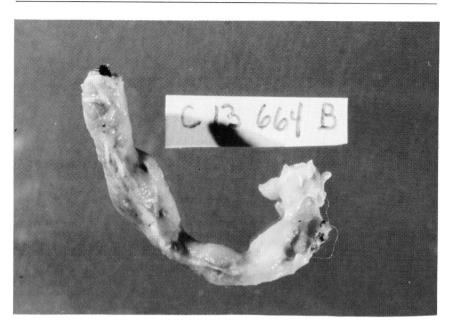

Figure 4. Atherosclerotic vein graft disease: macroscopic appearance. The graft shows gross atheromatous infiltration of vein wall.

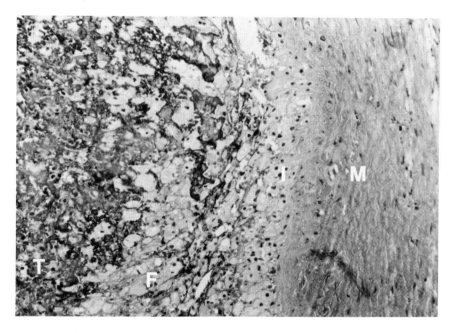

Figure 5. Atherosclerotic vein graft disease: microscopic aspect. Atheromatous foam cells (F) infiltrate and cover the intima (I) and the graft is completely obliterated by a thrombus (T). The media (M) is normal.

79% at one year, and 78% at three years. Another group of 108 patients underwent sequential angiography one and six years after surgery. Between the two studies, 17 of the 159 grafts became occluded, for an attrition rate of 11% over the five-year period.

In a further evaluation of 132 vein grafts that were patent at one year in 82 patients, 30% of the grafts had become occluded at 10 to 12 years, evidence of atherosclerotic disease in patent grafts was found in 33% and only 37% of the grafts had retained a normal angiographic appearance.[55] Among this group, iterative angiographic examination was performed 1, 5 to 7, and 10 to 12 years after operation, in 60 patients (Figure 3). Graft patency rates were 90, 80, and 60% respectively. At one year, no evidence of atherosclerotic graft disease was found, but it was present in 13 and in 27% of the grafts at the second and third evaluation. Therefore, after 10 years, atherosclerosis had developed in nearly half of the vein grafts that were still patent. Very similar rates of patency and of vein graft disease were found in other studies at 1,[56] 5,[57] and between 5 and 10 years after operation.[58]

Pathologic examination of venous grafts available from autopsy or reoperation has shown three different mechanisms of graft occlusion.[54] In the first month following operation, occlusion was almost always due to graft thrombosis which was related to surgical technique. Graft occlusions between one month and one year were due to intimal proliferation of smooth muscle cells with medial fibrosis. It was stipulated that intimal fibrous hyperplasia was the result of a repair response of the saphenous vein wall to surgical manipulations and to ischemia caused by dissection and isolation of the vein. Graft atherosclerosis as a cause of occlusion was never present during the first two years, but it was found in 42% of vein grafts examined after 24 months (Figures 4 & 5). In fact, late graft modifications, which appear after the first year, are always due to atherosclerotic vein graft disease.[32]

VEIN GRAFT DISEASE

In a study of accelerated atherosclerosis in saphenous vein grafts, it was suggested that the early intimal thickening of the vein wall might play a role in the atherosclerotic process, through the formation of fibrous plaques which exhibited changes characteristic of atheroma.[59] However, by comparing sequential angiograms in the same patients, a similar prevalence of atherosclerosis at 10 to 12 years was found in grafts that were normal and in those with diffuse narrowing at the 6- to 18-month study.[55] The lack of correlation between angiographic evidence of early intimal fibrous hyperplasia and late atherosclerotic vein graft disease suggested that other mechanisms were involved. No correlation was found with patient age, extent of coronary artery disease and the usual common risk factors. However, patients with vein graft disease had a significantly higher low-density lipoprotein serum level and a lower high-density lipoprotein level than those without graft atherosclerosis.[55,60]

PROGRESSION OF DISEASE IN NATIVE CIRCULATION

Progression in the extent and severity of coronary artery disease has been found at angiograms performed 10 to 12 years after operation.[32] Significant changes had occurred in 47% of ungrafted arteries, in 61% of those with patent grafts, and in 94% of coronary vessels with an occluded graft. Most often the changes in grafted vessels occurred proximal to the coronary anastomosis and evolved to complete occlusion. Whereas the difference in disease progression between grafted and ungrafted arteries was not significant, it was significantly greater in those coronary vessels with occluded vein grafts.[60] The rate of progression was not related to age, sex, risk factors or extent of coronary disease at preoperative angiography. As in vein graft disease, high-density lipoprotein level was significantly lower and low-density lipoprotein significantly higher in patients with progression of disease in nongrafted coronary arteries. Patients who developed new lesions either in the native circulation or in vein grafts had significantly higher levels of total cholesterol, triglyceride, low-density lipoprotein cholesterol and low-density lipoprotein apoprotein B, and a lower level of high-density lipoprotein cholesterol than patients without progression of the disease.[61] It can therefore be concluded that atherosclerosis of both vein graft and native circulation is a progressive disease that is mainly related to plasma lipoprotein levels. The loss of clinical improvement with time correlates directly with the progression of atherosclerosis in vein grafts and in the native coronary circulation.[31]

PREVENTION AND TREATMENT OF VEIN GRAFT OCCLUSION AND ATHEROSCLEROTIC DISEASE

ANTIPLATELET THERAPY

In 1982, a study from the Mayo Clinic[62] reported that a combination of dipyridamole and aspirin therapy, started before and continued after aortocoronary bypass grafting, decreased graft occlusion significantly after operation. In 1984, this group indicated that the same antiplatelet regimen also decreased the one-year graft occlusion rate.[63] While the one-month occlusion rate was 2% in the treatment group compared to 10% in the control group, the cumulative rates were 11 and 23% respectively after a median of one year. It was hypothesized that platelet inhibitor therapy prevented the early platelet thrombotic occlusion of the grafts as well as the late phase of occlusion due to platelet thrombosis on intimal hyperplasia later on during the first year.[64] A study from a different group comparing the effect of low-dose aspirin alone with the association of aspirin and dipyridamole demonstrated to the superiority of the dual drug-therapy over control or aspirin alone in decreasing the occlusion rate at one month, from 18% in the placebo group to 14% in the aspirin-alone group, and 13% with the combined therapy.[65]

However, these results were disputed by others. In another randomized study, early graft patency improved with platelet inhibitor therapy started early (second day) after operation, and both aspirin alone and aspirin with dipyridamole were equally effective.[66] The need to initiate the treatment preoperatively and to associate the two drugs was therefore questioned. A Veterans Administration Cooperative Study[67] investigated a number of antiplatelet therapy regimens started preoperatively. All treatment regimens improved early graft patency within two months of surgery from 85% in control patients to between 90 and 93% in treated groups. The results with aspirin alone once a day were as good as those with aspirin three times daily, aspirin and dipyridamole and sulfinpyrazone. However, all aspirin-containing regimens also increased postoperative bleeding and mediastinal reexploration compared with the nonaspirin groups. The fate of vein grafts was restudied after one year by the same group.[68] The one-year cumulative graft occlusion rate was 16% in all aspirin groups combined and 23% in the placebo group. This significant difference at one year disappeared when occlusions that occurred within the first two months were excluded, thus suggesting that aspirin might not improve the patency rate of vein grafts after the early postoperative period of two to three months. This subject thus remains controversial, hence the conflicting opinions regarding the duration of treatment with aspirin after operation. It is not yet clearly established whether platelets play a role in the development of atherosclerotic vein graft disease or not, but if they do, long-term platelet inhibitor therapy might then be beneficial.

CONTROL OF PLASMA LIPIDS

Several studies have shown a close correlation between vein graft disease and plasma lipid levels.[58,60,61,69] Control of all risk factors for coronary artery disease appears mandatory to decrease the progression of coronary disease and the development of vein graft disease, particularly that of dyslipidemia which is a frequent finding in patients undergoing coronary bypass grafting. New

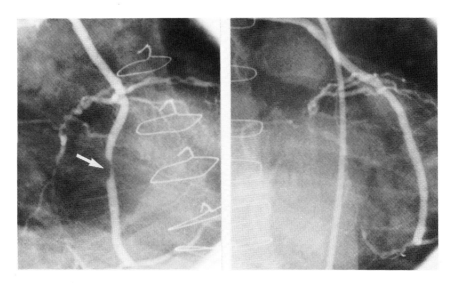

Figure 6. Angiogram of saphenous vein graft 13 years after coronary artery bypass grafting in an elderly patient, showing severe narrowing of mid-portion of graft (arrow) due to atherosclerotic disease (left). After angioplasty, the stenosis is completely relieved (right). Angioplasty was chosen rather than surgery because of advanced age and poor general condition of this patient, and because of the presence of three other normal vein grafts.

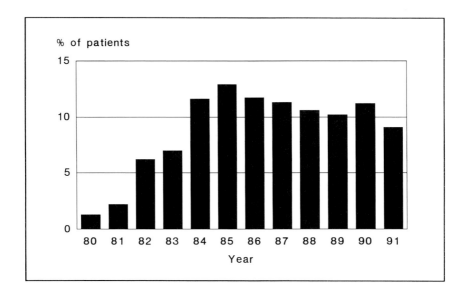

Figure 7. Ratio of reoperations for myocardial revascularization among patients undergoing coronary artery bypass grafting each year at the Montreal Heart Institute (range of total number of patients per year: from 542 in 1980 to 984 in 1991).

lipid-reducing drugs are effective and usually well tolerated.[70,71] This, along with a low-lipid diet, may help to improve late clinical outcome of surgery and prevent or postpone the need for reoperation.[72,73] In a case control study from the Milwaukee Cardiovascular Data Registry,[74] the 166 male patients who underwent repeat coronary grafting had a significantly higher triglyceride serum level than the 428 patients who had a single procedure. In this study the triglyceride level was the strongest predictor of reoperation, thus suggesting that lipid-lowering treatment may effectively reduce significantly the risk of progression of the disease in native coronary vessels and in vein grafts.

ANGIOPLASTY OF DISEASED VEIN GRAFTS

In well-selected cases, angioplasty of diseased vein grafts or of anastomotic stenoses may be a valuable alternative treatment to reoperation. The success rate is excellent for all sites of dilatations whether at proximal or distal anastomoses, or at the body of the graft itself.[75,76] The lesion can be successfully dilated in 85% of the patients. However, there is a high rate of restenosis, between 35 and 65%, particularly at aortic anastomoses and in the body of the graft. Older grafts have a greater tendency to restenosis. In addition, the complication rate is not negligible, with a 5% myocardial infarction rate, a 2% rate of emergent surgery, and a 1% mortality.

The role of angioplasty in the treatment of atherosclerotic graft disease, for lesions in the body of the graft, is limited to disabled patients who are not suitable for surgery because of advanced age, poor general condition, severe myocardial dysfunction or inoperable coronary disease (Figure 6). The decision to offer angioplasty must be weighed against the high recurrence rate in this particular location and the risk of embolization of atheromatous debris during the procedure. On the contrary, patients with anastomotic stenoses, particularly at the distal end, are good candidates for angioplasty in order to avoid reoperation. Dilatation of stenoses at the coronary anastomosis has a long-term patency rate greater than 90%.[76]

REOPERATION FOR VEIN GRAFT DISEASE AND OCCLUSION

In our experience, the number of patients undergoing reoperation for coronary artery bypass grafting has increased markedly from 1980 to 1985, when it reached a peak with 101 procedures during that year, or 13% of the patients undergoing myocardial revascularization. Since then, the ratio of reoperations tends to decrease yearly, to just about 9% of all coronary bypass cases in 1991 (Figure 7).

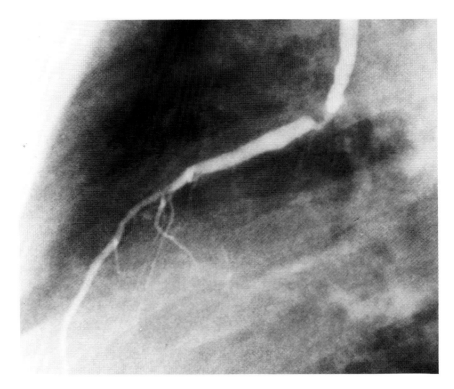

Figure 8. Angiogram of saphenous vein graft 15 years after operation showing severe mid-portion stenosis, in a patient who underwent reoperation.

Indications for reoperation vary according to the time period between the initial and the second operation. Reoperation during the first month following initial operation is usually due to early thrombosis of the graft which is always related to technical factors. Between one month and one year, graft occlusion because of intimal fibrous hyperplasia is nearly always the cause for reoperation. These two events which used to be more frequent in the early days of coronary artery bypass grafting are now rarely seen. Between one and six years, progression of the disease in the native circulation is the main indication for reoperation. None of the preceding situations present a particular problem at reoperation, except for the risk of resternotomy, which can be minimized by lifting the sternum with the untwisted stainless steel wires during the sternotomy with the oscillating saw.

After the sixth year, reoperation poses a completely different challenge, with significantly higher mortality and complication rates.[77] The increased risk has been attributed to the fact that vein graft disease is the main cause for reoperation in these patients (Figure 8). Atherosclerotic grafts contain friable atheroma and thrombotic debris that may be a source of embolization to

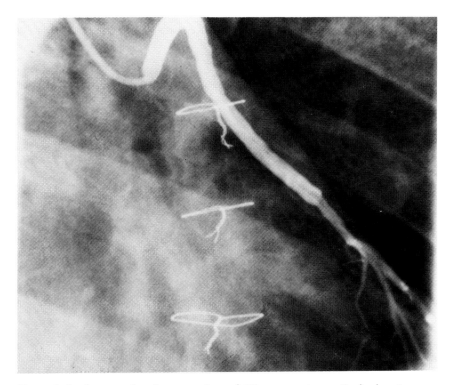

Figure 9. Angiogram of saphenous vein graft 15 years postoperatively showing near normal vein graft. At reoperation for progression of disease in native coronary arteries, moderate diffuse atheromatous infiltration of vein wall was found, and the graft was replaced.

distal coronary arteries during surgery.[78] A different surgical approach has been proposed in order to decrease the risk of perioperative myocardial infarction and death due to atheromatous embolization.[79] Initial experience with early ligation of all patent grafts and construction of all distal and proximal anastomoses during a single period of aortic cross-clamping in a small number of patients had suggested an improvement in surgical results, with a decrease in morbidity and mortality. However, further experience in a larger group of patients has shown that the risk of reoperation remained considerably higher than that of first operation, despite the use of such precautions. In a group of 331 patients who underwent reoperation between 1984 and 1989, after an average of nearly nine years following initial operation, the early mortality was 12% and the myocardial infarction rate 18%.[80] This was considerably higher than the 2% mortality and the 3% perioperative myocardial infarction rates observed among patients who underwent surgery for the first time during the same period. In a previous study from the CASS registry,[81] it had been reported that reoperation performed after an average of

Table 2. Surgical Mortality and Myocardial Infarction Rates Among 321 Patients Undergoing Reoperation for Coronary Artery Bypass Grafting, from 19 to 212 Months (mean: 106 months) after Initial Operation. Data from Perrault and coll.[85]

	No. of patients	Operative mortality (%)	Myocardial infarction (%)
Status of Vein Graft:			
all grafts normal or occluded	82	7*	11*
one atheromatous graft	142	7*	12*
two atheromatous grafts	69	17*	29*
three atheromatous grafts	28	29*	32*
Surgical Technique for Atheromatous Grafts:			
grafts ligated and single aortic cross-clamping	66	17†	23†
grafts ligated and two aortic clampings	35	9†	17†
no early ligation of grafts and two aortic clampings	138	12†	18†

* p < 0.01; † differences not significant (p > 0.05).

just over three years following initial surgery carried a risk of mortality only slightly higher than the first operation (5.3% versus 3.1%), and a rate of myocardial infarction which was not significantly different (6.4% versus 5.9%). From these two studies, it appears obvious that the two patient populations had a very different risk profile, related to the interval period between the two procedures, and hence to the underlying disease process.

In a comparative analysis of 6591 primary operations and 508 reoperations, the change in risk with the interval between the two procedures was clearly demonstrated.[82] Whereas the operative mortality of primary operation was 2%, that of reoperation within one year of first procedure was 3.6%, between 1 and 5 years 5.9%, 6% from 5 to 10 years, and 17.6% after 10 years. The overall myocardial infarction rate of 9% at reoperation was significantly higher than the rate of 4% at primary surgery. However, multiple reoperation procedures do not appear to increase the risk any further.[83] Replacing all previous vein grafts, including those that look normal at angiography (Figure 9), and a more extensive use of internal mammary grafts at the second operation may decrease the need for a third operation by 20% or more.[84]

A study of risk factors among our patients who underwent reoperation showed that at age 60 years or older, preoperative unstable angina or recent myocardial infarction and atherosclerotic patent saphenous vein grafts were significant predictors of early mortality, whereas only the latter was a significant risk factor for perioperative myocardial infarction.[80] A more comprehensive evaluation of the significance of atheromatous vein graft disease indicated a positive correlation between early mortality at reoperation and the number of patent diseased vein grafts.[85] The mortality was 7% with one, 17% with two, and 29% with three or more patent atheromatous grafts. The surgical technique used at reoperation, whether the grafts had been ligated early during operation or not, and a single aortic cross-clamping period had been used or not for all distal and proximal anastomoses, had no significant effect on the mortality rate. Results with regard to the incidence of perioperative myocardial infarction were similar. A direct positive correlation was found with the number of diseased grafts, with respective infarction rates of 12, 29, and 32%, whereas the surgical approach had no significant influence (Table 2).

Two mechanisms are probably involved in the increased morbidity and mortality of reoperation for atheromatous vein grafts. Embolization of atheromatous debris remains the dominant threat, but our experience has shown that the modifications in surgical technique proposed so far have failed to improve the results significantly. This may be due to the difficulty of achieving adequate and even delivery of cardioplegic solution to all myocardial areas when patent vein grafts are interrupted at the beginning of the procedure. Therefore, one is caught between the choice of better myocardial protection at the risk of atheromatous embolization, or prevention of the latter at the expense of the former. Retrograde infusion of blood cardioplegia through the coronary sinus may be the proper answer to this problem. Retrograde cardioplegia has been shown to be as effective as the antegrade administration route and to provide excellent myocardial protection and postoperative functional recovery in patients undergoing coronary artery bypass grafting.[86] In reoperations, it would provide a more even distribution of cardioplegia to the myocardium, while at the same time it would wash out from the coronary arteries through the grafts the atheromatous debris that may have been dislodged during surgical manipulations. However, this hypothesis remains to be tested in a prospective randomized trial.

Late survival following reoperation is 90% at 5 years and 75% at 10 years.[87] Long-term survival of patients who left hospital after reoperation is similar to that following primary operation, although event-free survival is slightly lower.[82] Advanced age, hypertension and abnormal left ventricular function have been identified as significant predictors of decreased late survival.[87]

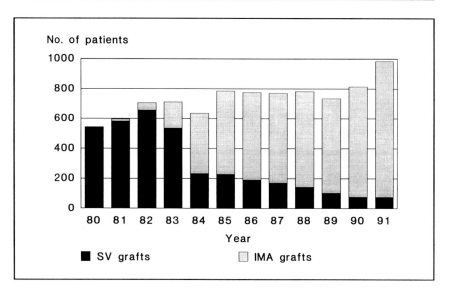

Figure 10. Number of patients in whom saphenous vein (SV) grafts only were used, and number of those with at least one internal mammary artery (IMA) graft, each year from 1980 to 1991, at the Montreal Heart Institute.

CURRENT TRENDS IN MYOCARDIAL REVASCULARIZATION

CHANGES IN PATIENT POPULATION

A progressive change in the population of patients undergoing myocardial revascularization over the years has been well documented. During the first decade of aortocoronary bypass grafting, there had been a gradual decrease in early mortality and in perioperative myocardial infarction rate, despite the fact that patients in the period after 1975 had a more severe coronary artery disease and a slightly more frequent abnormal left ventricular function[88,89] The improvement in results had been attributed to increased surgical experience, improved myocardial protection, and more complete myocardial revascularization. The lowest early mortality and infarction rates have been achieved in the early 1980's, with respective rates of 1%, and 2 to 4%.[24,88,89]

However, after 1985, a significant rise in the operative risk of myocardial revascularization was observed in most centers. Increases in mortality rates to between 5 and 8% were reported, along with increases in the need for postoperative mechanical support and in myocardial infarction rate to more than 5% each.[90,91] Beside the extent and severity of coronary involvement, several other factors have contributed to change the profile of the surgical patients. There was a marked increase in the number of patients older than 70 years of age, with various associated physical conditions, particularly renal, pulmonary and vascular dysfunctions as well as cerebrovascular disease. Noncardiac complications are the main cause of postoperative morbidity and mortality in this age group.[51] Congestive heart failure and severe left ventricular dysfunction were more common in surgical patients in recent years. A more aggressive attitude in the treatment of these patients has developed as a result of the data indicating that late survival was particularly improved in this subset, and with the improvement in myocardial protection during surgery, and better circulatory support and care during the immediate postoperative period.

The success of coronary angioplasty has had a major impact on the changing characteristics of the surgical patient. Angioplasty is successful in about two-thirds of the patients, with a low morbidity and mortality, although recurrences occur in approximately 25% of the patients.[92] As a result, patients with single-vessel disease are not directed toward surgical treatment any more, and this low-risk patient has proportionally vanished from surgical series.[93] On the other hand, acute coronary occlusion complicating coronary angioplasty has contributed its share of high-risk patients to surgical treatment. This complication is more common in patients with unstable angina, multivessel disease and complex coronary artery lesions.[94] Perioperative morbidity and mortality are significantly higher following complicated coronary angioplasty, particularly when the patient has to undergo urgent or emergent surgery.[95,96]

Finally, the increasing number of reoperations has also been responsible in part for the higher risk and complication rate of myocardial revascularization in recent years.[80,82,85] In addition to the risk of coronary embolization, these patients often come to surgery in a worse clinical condition because of unstable angina, recent myocardial infarction and extensive coronary artery disease.[97] However, there are indications that the number of reoperations may now be on a slightly decreasing slope, probably as a result of the more extensive use of arterial conduits at primary operations.

CHANGES IN OPERATIVE APPROACH

Whereas saphenous vein grafts were used in 100% of our patients in 1980, the use of internal mammary artery grafts has progressively gained in popularity, and, since 1986, the latter has been used for at least one graft in more than 75% of patients each year (Figure 10). In 1991, the proportion of patients in whom an arterial conduit was used was up to 92% (908/984 patients), and nearly 50% of all coronary grafts were constructed with the internal mammary artery (1376/2792 grafts). Our experience is similar to that of many other centers. This shift away from vein grafts and toward arterial grafts occurred as a result of comparative studies indicating that the latter had a much better long-term prognosis than the former, and remained free from atherosclerotic disease up to 10 years, leading to a better 10-year survival.[58,98,99] It is now generally accepted that the internal mammary artery is the graft of choice for coronary bypass grafting.[100] In recent years, other arterial conduits have also been evaluated. We have used the right gastroepiploic artery in selected patients since 1989, and the inferior epigastric artery in a small series since 1991. These various arterial conduits and their results will be discussed in further chapters.

Finally, myocardial protection has been another area of major change in later years, with the shift from cold crystalloid cardioplegia, to cold blood and more recently to warm blood cardioplegia. Better myocardial protection during surgery has improved the results in more diseased and higher risk patients and has opened the way to new indications for coronary artery bypass grafting in patients who were formerly considered inoperable.

CONCLUSION

The large multicenter randomized studies have played a determinant role in the definition of more precise indications for surgical revascularization of the myocardium. However, since then, the advent of coronary angioplasty has modified the profile of patients currently undergoing surgical treatment. On the other hand, the serial angiographic evaluations of vein and arterial grafts have determined the respective durability of these conduits, establishing without any doubt the superiority of arterial grafts over vein grafts at 10 years. With our better understanding of the pathophysiology of vein graft disease, preventive measures now appear as an essential step in improving the durability of vein grafts.

Because of the very large population of patients with vein grafts implanted more than seven years ago, the incidence of reoperation for vein graft disease, with its higher complication and mortality rates, will remain a major issue, even though the number of second operations may now appear to be on the downward slope, as a result of the more extensive use of arterial grafts in latter years. Nevertheless, vein grafts will continue to occupy a major place in coronary artery bypass grafting, although they have evolved to a more adjuvant role, as conduits for smaller or less important coronary arteries, while arterial conduits are routinely used for coronary territories of greater significance. Further improvements in late clinical results and graft patency can be foreseen with the use of arterial grafts in a large majority of patients. This may be particularly significant in younger patients with dyslipidemia and severe coronary artery disease in whom the choice of arterial conduits is essential, as is the adequate control of the various risk factors including hyperlipidemia, tobacco, hypertension and life style, if long-lasting results are to be expected.

REFERENCES

1. Carrel A. On the experimental surgery of the thoracic aorta and heart. Ann Surg 1910; 52:83-95.

2. Beck CS, Tietry VL, Moretz AR. Production of a collateral circulation to the heart. Proc Soc Exp Biol Med 1935; 32:759-61.

3. Vineberg AM, Miller WD. An experimental study of the physiological role of the anastomosis between the left coronary circulation and left internal mammary artery implanted in the left ventricular myocardium. Surg Forum 1950; 5:294-9.

4. Murray G, Porcheron R, Hilario J et al. Anastomosis of a systemic artery to the coronary. Can Med Ass J 1954; 71:594-7.

5. Thal A, Perry JF Jr, Miller FA et al. Direct suture anastomosis of the coronary arteries in the dog. Surgery 1956; 40:1023-9.

6. Sones FM Jr, Shirey EK. Cine coronary arteriography. Mod Conc Cardiovasc Dis 1962; 3:735-8.

7. Senning A. Strip grafting in coronary arteries. Report of a case. J Thorac Cardiovasc Surg 1961; 41:542-9.

8. Effler DB, Sones FM Jr, Favaloro R et al. Coronary endarterotomy with patch-graft reconstruction: Clinical experience with 34 cases. Ann Surg 1965; 162:590-601.

9. Garrett HE, Dennis EW, DeBakey ME. Aortocoronary bypass with saphenous vein graft. JAMA 1973; 223:792-4.

10. Favaloro RG. Saphenous vein autograft replacement of severe segmental coronary artery occlusion. Operative technique. Ann Thorac Surg 1968; 5:334-9.

11. Johnson WD, Lepley D Jr. An aggressive surgical approach to coronary disease. J Thorac Cardiovasc Surg 1970; 59:128-38.

12. Saltiel J, Lespérance J, Bourassa MG et al. Reversibility of left ventricular dysfunction following aortocoronary bypass grafts. Am J Roentgen Rad Ther Nucl Med 1970; 110:739-46.

13. Kolessov VI. Mammary artery-coronary artery anastomosis as method of treatment for angina pectoris. J Thorac Cardiovasc Surg 1967; 54:535-44.

14. Green GE, Stertzer SH, Reppert EH. Coronary arterial bypass grafts. Ann Thorac Surg 1968; 5:443-50.

15. Green GE, Stertzer SH, Gordon RB et al. Anastomosis of the internal mammary artery to the distal left anterior descending coronary artery. Circulation 1970; 41(suppl II):II-79-II-85.

16. Loop FD, Effler DB, Spampinato N et al. Myocardial revascularization by internal mammary artery grafts. A technique without optical assistance. J Thorac Cardiovasc Surg 1972; 63:674-80.

17. Hultgren HN, Detre KM, Takaro T et al. The VA Cooperative Study of coronary arterial surgery: Baseline characteristics of study population and survival in subgroups with medical versus surgical treatment. In: Yu PN, Goodwin JF, eds. Progress in Cardiology, vol. 6, Philadelphia: Lea & Febiger 1977:67-81.

18. Varnaukas E, Olsson SB. The European Multicenter CABG Trial. In: Yu PN, Goodwin JF, eds. Progress in Cardiology, vol. 6, Philadelphia: Lea & Febiger 1977:83-9.

19. Principal Investigators of CASS and their Associates (Killip T, Fisher LD, Mock MB, eds.) National Heart, Lung, and Blood Institute Coronary Artery Surgery Study (CASS). Circulation 1981; 63(suppl I):I-1-I-81.

20. Fisher LD, Davis KB. Design and study similarities and contrasts: The Veterans Administration, European, and CASS randomized trials of coronary artery bypass graft surgery. Circulation 1985; 72 (suppl V):V-110-V-6.

21. Bristow JD. A cardiologist's view of coronary bypass surgery. In: Yu PN, Goodwin JF, eds. Progress in Cardiology, vol. 6, Philadelphia: Lea & Febiger 1977:1-40.

22. Guiteras Val P, Pelletier LC, Galinanes Hernandez M et al. Diagnostic criteria and prognosis of perioperative myocardial infarction following coronary bypass. J Thorac Cardiovasc Surg 1983; 86:878-86.

23. Cosgrove DM, Loop FD, Lytle BW et al. Primary myocardial revascularization. Trends in surgical mortality. J Thorac Cardiovasc Surg 1984; 88:673-84.

24. Ennabli K, Pelletier LC. Evaluation de la protection myocardique dans le pontage aorto-coronarien. Coeur 1985; 16:589-95.

25. Bourassa MG. Long-term clinical results after coronary artery bypass surgery. In: Waters DD, Bourassa MG, eds. Care of the Patient With Previous Coronary Bypass Surgery. Brest AN, ed. Cardiovascular Clinics, vol. 21, Philadelphia: FA Davis 1991:101-21.

26. Kaiser GC, Davis KB, Fisher LD et al. Survival following coronary artery bypass grafting in patients with severe angina pectoris (CASS). J Thorac Cardiovasc Surg 1985; 89:513-24.

27. Alderman EL, Fisher LD, Litwin P et al. Results of coronary artery surgery in patients with poor left ventricular function (CASS). Circulation 1983; 68:785-95.

28. Varnauskas E, and the European Coronary Surgery Study Group. Twelve-year follow-up of survival in the randomized European Coronary Surgery Study. N Engl J Med 1988; 319:332-7.

29. Alderman EL, Bourassa MG, Cohen LS et al. Ten-year follow-up of survival and myocardial infarction in the randomized Coronary Artery Surgery Study. Circulation 1990; 82:1629-46.

30. Veterans Administration Coronary Artery Bypass Surgery Cooperative Study Group. Eleven-year survival in the Veterans Administration randomized trial of coronary bypass surgery for stable angina. N Engl J Med 1984; 311:1333-9.

31. Campeau L, Lespérance J, Hermann J et al. Loss of improvement of angina between 1 and 7 years after aortocoronary bypass surgery. Correlations with changes in vein grafts and in coronary arteries. Circulation 1979; 60(suppl I):I-1-I-5.

32. Campeau L, Bourassa MG, Enjalbert M et al. Improvement of angina and survival 1 to 12 years after aortocoronary bypass surgery: Correlations with changes in grafts and in the native coronary circulation. J Heart Transplant 1984; 3:220-3.

33. CASS Principal Investigators and their Associates. Coronary Artery Surgery Study (CASS): A randomized trial of coronary artery bypass surgery. Quality of life in patients randomly assigned to treatment groups. Circulation 1983; 68:951-60.

34. Rogers WJ, Coggin CJ, Gersh BJ et al. Ten-year follow-up of quality of life in patients randomized to receive medical therapy or coronary artery bypass graft surgery. The Coronary Artery Surgery Study (CASS). Circulation 1990; 82:1647-58.

35. Varnauskas E, and the European Coronary Surgery Study Group. Survival, myocardial infarction, and employment status in a prospective randomized study of coronary bypass surgery. Circulation 1985; 72(suppl V):V-90-V-101.

36. Danchin N, David P, Bourassa MG et al. Factors predicting working status after aortocoronary bypass surgery. Can Med Assoc J 1982; 126:255-60.

37. Boulay FM, David PP, Bourassa MG. Strategies for improving the work status of patients after coronary artery bypass surgery. Circulation 1982; 66(suppl III):III-43-III-9.

38. Detre KM, Takaro T, Hultgren H et al. Long-term mortality and morbidity results of the Veterans Administration randomized trial of coronary artery bypass surgery. Circulation 1985; 72(suppl V):V-84-V-9.

39. Bourassa MG. Left ventricular function after coronary bypass surgery. In: Waters DD, Bourassa MG, eds. Care of the Patient With Previous Coronary Bypass Surgery. Brest AN, ed. Cardiovascular Clinics, vol. 21, Philadelphia: FA Davis 1991:227-37.

40. Campeau L, Corbara F, Crochet D et al. Left main coronary artery stenosis. The influence of aortocoronary bypass surgery on survival. Circulation 1978; 57:1111-5.

41. Takaro T, Peduzzi P, Detre KM et al. Survival in subgroups of patients with left main coronary artery disease. Veterans Administration Cooperative Study of surgery for coronary arterial occlusive disease. Circulation 1982; 66:14-22.

42. Golding LAR, Loop FD, Sheldon WC et al. Emergency revascularization for unstable angina. Circulation 1978; 58:1163-6.

43. Akins CW. Indications and results of surgery in unstable angina and Prinzmetal's variant angina. In: McGoon D, ed. Cardiac Surgery. Cardiovascular Clinics, vol. 12, Brest AN, ed. Philadelphia: FA Davis 1982:49-59.

44. Théroux P, Ouimet H, McCans J et al. Aspirin, heparin, or both to treat acute unstable angina. N Engl J Med 1988; 319:1105-11.

45. Parasi AF, Khuri S, Deupree RH et al. Medical compared with surgical management of unstable angina: 5-year mortality and morbidity in the Veterans Administration Study. Circulation 1989; 80:1176-89.

46. Berg R Jr, Selinger SL, Leonard JJ et al. Immediate coronary artery bypass for acute evolving myocardial infarction. J Thorac Cardiovasc Surg 1981; 81:493-7.

47. Théroux P, Waters DD, Halphen C et al. Prognostic value of exercise testing soon after myocardial infarction. N Engl J Med 1979; 301:341-5.

48. Jones EL, Waites TF, Craver JM et al. Coronary bypass for relief of persistent pain following acute myocardial infarction. Ann Thorac Surg 1981; 32:33-43.

49. Grondin CM, Kretz JG, Vouhé P et al. Prophylactic coronary artery grafting in patients with few or no symptoms. Ann Thorac Surg 1979; 28:113-8.

50. CASS Principal Investigators and their Associates. Myocardial infarction and mortality in the Coronary Artery Surgery Study (CASS) randomized trial. N Engl J Med 1984; 310:750-8.

51. Ennabli K, Pelletier LC. Morbidity and mortality of coronary artery surgery after the age of 70 years. Ann Thorac Surg 1986; 42:197-200.

52. Horvath KA, DiSesa VJ, Peigh PS et al. Favorable results of coronary artery bypass grafting in patients older than 75 years. J Thorac Cardiovasc Surg 1990; 99:92-6.

53. Bourassa MG, Fisher LD, Campeau L et al. Long-term fate of bypass grafts: The Coronary Artery Surgery Study (CASS) and Montreal Heart Institute experiences. Circulation 1985; 72(suppl V):V-71-V-8.

54. Bourassa MG, Campeau L, Lespérance J et al. Changes in grafts and coronary arteries after saphenous vein aortocoronary bypass surgery: Results at repeat angiography. Circulation 1982; 65(suppl II):II-90-II-7.

55. Campeau L, Enjalbert M, Lespérance J et al. Atherosclerosis and late closure of aortocoronary saphenous vein grafts: Sequential angiographic studies at 2 weeks, 1 year, 5 to 7 years, and 10 to 12 years after surgery. Circulation 1983; 68(suppl II):II-1-II-7.

56. FitzGibbon GM, Burton JR, Leach AJ. Coronary bypass graft fate: Angiographic grading of 1400 consecutive grafts early after operation and of 1132 after one year. Circulation 1978; 57:1070-4.

57. FitzGibbon GM, Leach AJ, Keon WJ et al. Coronary bypass graft fate: Angiographic study of 1179 vein grafts early, one year, and five years after operation. J Thorac Cardiovasc Surg 1986; 91:773-8.

58. Lytle BW, Loop FD, Cosgrove DM et al. Long-term (5 to 12 years) serial studies of internal mammary artery and saphenous vein coronary bypass grafts. J Thorac Cardiovasc Surg 1985; 89:248-58.

59. Bulkley BH, Hutchins GM. Accelerated "atherosclerosis": A morphologic study of 97 saphenous vein coronary artery bypass grafts. Circulation 1977; 55:163-8.

60. Bourassa MG, Enjalbert M, Campeau L et al. Progression of atherosclerosis in coronary arteries and bypass grafts: Ten years later. Am J Cardiol 1984; 53:102C-7C.

61. Campeau L, Enjalbert M, Lespérance J et al. The relation of risk factors to the development of atherosclerosis in saphenous-vein bypass grafts and the progression of disease in the native circulation: A study 10 years after aortocoronary bypass surgery. N Engl J Med 1984; 311:1329-32.

62. Chesebro JH, Clements IP, Fuster V et al. A platelet-inhibitor-drug trial in coronary-artery bypass operations: Benefit of perioperative dipyridamole and aspirin therapy on early postoperative vein-graft patency. N Engl J Med 1982; 307:73-8.

63. Chesebro JH, Fuster V, Elveback LR et al. Effect of dipyridamole and aspirin on late vein-graft patency after coronary bypass operations. N Engl J Med 1984; 310:209-14.

64. Fuster V, Chesebro JH. Role of platelets and platelet inhibitors in aortocoronary artery vein-graft disease. Circulation 1986; 73:227-32.

65. Sanz G, Pajaron A, Alegria E et al. Prevention of early aortocoronary bypass occlusion by low-dose aspirin and dipyridamole. Circulation 1990; 82:765-73.

66. Brown BG, Cukingnan RA, DeRouen T et al. Improved graft patency in patients treated with platelet-inhibiting therapy after coronary bypass surgery. Circulation 1985; 72:138-46.

67. Goldman S, Copeland J, Moritz T et al. Improvement in early saphenous vein graft patency after coronary artery bypass surgery with antiplatelet therapy: Results of a Veterans Administration Cooperative Study. Circulation 1988; 77:1324-32.

68. Goldman S, Copeland J, Moritz T et al. Saphenous vein graft patency 1 year after coronary artery bypass surgery and effects of antiplatelet therapy: Results of a Veterans Administration Cooperative Study. Circulation 1989; 80:1190-7.

69. Solymoss BC, Leung TK, Pelletier LC et al. Pathologic changes in coronary artery saphenous vein grafts and related etiologic factors. In: Waters DD, Bourassa MG, eds. Care of the Patient With Previous Coronary Bypass Surgery. Cardiovascular Clinics, vol. 21, Brest AN, ed. Philadelphia: FA Davis, 1991:45-65.

70. Tobert JA. New developments in lipid-lowering therapy: The role of inhibitors of hydroxymethylglutarylcoenzyme A reductase. Circulation 1987; 76:534-8.

71. Lovastatin Study Group III. A multicenter comparison of lovastatin and cholestyramine therapy for severe primary hypercholesterolemia. JAMA 1988; 260:359-66.

72. Grundy SM. Dietary therapy for different forms of hyperlipoproteinemia. Circulation 1987; 76:523-8.

73. Tikkanen MJ, Nikkila EA. Current pharmacologic treatment of elevated serum cholesterol. Circulation 1987; 76:529-33.

74. Fox MH, Gruchow HW, Barboriak JJ et al. Risk factors among patients undergoing repeat aorta-coronary bypass procedures. J Thorac Cardiovasc Surg 1987; 93:56-61.

75. Côté G, Myler RK, Stertzer SH et al. Percutaneous transluminal angioplasty of stenotic coronary artery bypass grafts: 5-years' experience. J Am Coll Cardiol 1987; 9:8-17.

76. Reeves F, Bonan R, Côté G et al. Long-term angiographic follow-up after angioplasty of venous coronary bypass grafts. Am Heart J 1991; 122:620-7.

77. Pelletier LC, Carrier M. Early postoperative care and complications. In Waters DD, Bourassa MG, eds. Care of the Patient With Previous Coronary Bypass Surgery. Cardiovascular Clinics, vol. 21, Brest AN, ed. Philadelphia: FA Davis 1991:3-24.

78. Keon WJ, Heggtveit HA, Leduc J. Perioperative myocardial infarction caused by atheroembolism. J Thorac Cardiovasc Surg 1982; 84:849-55.

79. Grondin CM, Pomar JL, Hébert Y et al. Reoperation in patients with patent atherosclerotic coronary vein grafts: A different approach to a different disease. J Thorac Cardiovasc Surg 1984; 87:379-85.

80. Carrier M, Perrault L, Pelletier LC. Reoperation for coronary artery bypass grafting. In: Waters DD, Bourassa MG, eds. Care of the Patient With Previous Coronary Bypass Surgery. Cardiovascular Clinics, vol. 21, Brest AN, ed. Philadelphia: FA Davis 1991:257-63.

81. Foster ED, Fisher LD, Kaiser GC et al. Comparison of operative mortality and morbidity for initial and repeat coronary artery bypass grafting: The Coronary Artery Surgery Study (CASS) registry experience. Ann Thorac Surg 1984; 38:563-70.

82. Salomon NW, Page US, Bigelow JC et al. Reoperative coronary surgery: Comparative analysis of 6591 patients undergoing primary bypass and 508 patients undergoing reoperative coronary artery bypass. J Thorac Cardiovasc Surg 1990; 100:250-60.

83. Accola KD, Craver JM, Weintraub WS et al. Multiple reoperative coronary artery bypass grafting. Ann Thorac Surg 1991; 52:738-44.

84. Owen EW Jr, Schoettle GP Jr, Marotti AS et al. The third time coronary artery bypass graft: Is the risk justified? J Thorac Cardiovasc Surg 1990; 100:31-5.

85. Perrault L, Carrier M, Cartier R et al. Morbidity and mortality of reoperation for coronary artery bypass grafting: Significance of atheromatous vein grafts. Can J Cardiol 1991; 7:427-30.

86. Diehl JT, Eichhorn EJ, Konstam MA et al. Efficacy of retrograde coronary sinus cardioplegia in patients undergoing myocardial revascularization: A prospective randomized trial. Ann Thorac Surg 1988; 45:595-602.

87. Lytle BW, Loop FD, Cosgrove DM et al. Fifteen hundred coronary reoperations: Results and determinants of early and late survival. J Thorac Cardiovasc Surg 1987; 93:847-59.

88. Loop FD, Cosgrove DM, Lytle BW et al. An 11-year evolution of coronary arterial surgery (1967-1978). Ann Surg 1979; 190:444-55.

89. Miller DC, Stinson EB, Oyer PE et al. Discriminant analysis of the changing risks of coronary artery operations: 1971-1979. J Thorac Cardiovasc Surg 1983; 85:197-213.

90. Naunheim KS, Fiore AC, Wadley JJ et al. The changing profile of the patient undergoing coronary artery bypass surgery. J Am Coll Cardiol 1988; 11:494-8.

91. Jones EL, Weintraub WS, Craver JM et al. Coronary bypass surgery: Is the operation different today? J Thorac Cardiovasc Surg 1991; 101:108-15.

92. Bourassa MG, Wilson JW, Detre KM et al. Long-term follow-up of coronary angioplasty: The 1977-1981 National Heart, Lung, and Blood Institute registry. Eur Heart J 1989; 10(suppl G):36-41.

93. Davis PK, Parascandola SA, Miller CA et al. Mortality of coronary artery bypass grafting before and after the advent of angioplasty. Ann Thorac Surg 1989; 47:493-8.

94. de Feyter PJ, van den Brand M, Jaarman G et al. Acute coronary artery occlusion during and after percutaneous transluminal coronary angioplasty: Frequency, prediction, clinical course, management, and follow-up. Circulation 1991; 83:927-36.

95. Pelletier LC, Pardini A, Renkin J et al. Myocardial revascularization after failure of percutaneous transluminal coronary angioplasty. J Thorac Cardiovasc Surg 1985; 90:265-71.

96. Naunheim KS, Fiore AC, Fagan DC et al. Emergency coronary artery bypass grafting for failed angioplasty: Risk factors and outcome. Ann Thorac Surg 1989; 47:816-23.

97. Wiseman A, Waters DD, Walling A et al. Long-term prognosis after myocardial infarction in patients with previous coronary artery bypass surgery. J Am Coll Cardiol 1988; 12:873-80.

98. Grondin CM, Campeau L, Lespérance J et al. Comparison of late changes in internal mammary artery and saphenous vein grafts in two consecutive series of patients 10 years after operation. Circulation 1984; 70(suppl I):I-208-I-12.

99. Loop FD, Lytle BW, Cosgrove DM et al. Influence of the internal-mammary-artery graft on 10-year survival and other cardiac events. N Engl J Med 1986; 314:1-6.

100. Carrier M, Grondin CM, Pelletier LC. The internal mammary artery: The graft of choice for coronary artery bypass. In: Copeland JG, Goldman S, eds. Improving Results with Coronary Artery Bypass Grafting. State of the Art Reviews: Cardiac Surgery, vol. 1, no. 1, Philadelphia: Hanley & Belfus Inc. 1986:87-97.

CHAPTER 3

THE INTERNAL MAMMARY ARTERY: WHY IS IT THE GRAFT OF CHOICE?

Michel Carrier

O nly a handful of surgeons have been enthusiastic supporters of the use of the internal mammary artery in coronary artery grafting in the early days of the procedure in the 1970s. However, progressively the idea has gained in popularity as long-term results obtained with the most commonly used vein graft have failed to meet expectations, due to accelerated atherosclerosis. At the same time, results were slowly accumulating, indicating that the internal mammary artery stood the test of time and could be the answer to the negative late results of surgical treatment of coronary artery disease.

The experience of the Montreal Heart Institute with the use of the internal mammary artery will be reviewed, and the place of this conduit in the surgical treatment of coronary artery disease today, the surgical technique, and the clinical outcomes will be discussed in the light of the experience of others.

CLINICAL RESULTS

The internal mammary artery (IMA) has been recognized for sometime as the conduit of choice for myocardial revascularization because of the

Table 1. Late Survival and Angiographic Results After Single Internal Mammary Artery Grafting of LAD with LIMA

Authors	Year of Report	No. of Patients	No. of Grafts Studied	10-Year Patency Rate	10-Year Patient Survival
Grondin et al[1]	1984	20	16	94%	84%
Okie et al[8]	1984	259	31	69%	82%
Barner et al[9]	1985	1000	442	88%	84%
Olearchyk et al[10]	1986	833			89%
Loop et al[7]	1986	2306	23	96%	87%
Cameron et al[11]	1986	532			82%
Ivert et al[12]	1988	99	37*	88%	74%
Zeff et al[13]	1988	39	35†	95%	92%
Kirklin et al[14]	1989	4790			89%

LAD: left anterior descending coronary artery
LIMA: left internal mammary artery
* Studied at 11 years
† Studied at 8.9 years

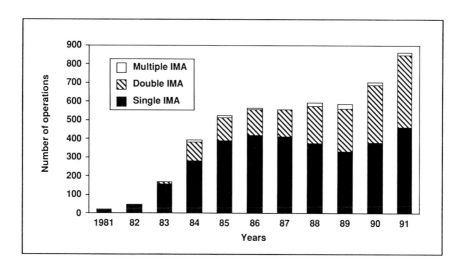

Figure 1. Number of patients who underwent coronary artery bypass grafting with single, double, and multiple internal mammary artery grafts, at the Montreal Heart Institute, from 1981 to 1991.

excellent long-term patency of the graft.[1-6] Moreover, Loop[7] and many other investigators[8-14] (Table 1) have found a significant improvement in the 10-year survival after IMA grafting to the anterior descending coronary artery, compared to patients with saphenous vein grafts. Failure to use an IMA graft to this coronary artery has been shown to be a risk factor for premature death, late myocardial infarction, recurrent hospitalization for cardiac events and for coronary reoperation.[6,7,14-18]

Today, guidelines for coronary artery grafting recommend the use of the left internal mammary artery graft to the anterior descending coronary artery in all patients, whenever feasible.[19-21] In our experience, the number of patients who underwent coronary artery bypass surgery with single or double internal mammary artery grafting has increased steadily between 1981 and 1991 (Figure 1).

EARLY MORBIDITY AND MORTALITY

In 1991, 45% of the patients undergoing myocardial revascularization at the Montreal Heart Institute had bilateral internal mammary artery grafting. However, despite its popularity, it has not yet been clearly established that bilateral mammary grafting improves long-term survival without also increasing the perioperative risk.[19]

From April 1991 to April 1992, 853 patients underwent elective or urgent coronary artery bypass grafting, among whom 400 had bilateral mammary artery grafting and 453 had single mammary artery grafts (Table 2). Patients with double internal mammary graft were significantly younger, had a smaller number of associated saphenous vein grafts, and were more likely to be males. Overall, perioperative mortality and morbidity rates were similar in both groups. There was a greater incidence of pleuropulmonary complications after surgery among patients with bilateral mammary grafting, mainly because of pleural effusion due to incidental pleurotomy at the time of internal mammary dissection. The incidence of wound infection was also higher after bilateral mammary grafting, but the difference was not statistically significant. Galbut and colleagues[22] reported perioperative mortality and morbidity rates similar to ours in patients with stable and unstable angina. The incidence of sternal wound infection was similarly low (1.5%), and diabetes was found to be a significant risk factor. In a controversial debate, Fiore and his group[23] initially suggested that patient survival at 15 years was better among patients who underwent double IMA grafting, compared to single IMA but, after obtaining a complete follow-up of their patients, they concluded that a significant effect on patient survival could not be demonstrated.[24] On the other hand, it has been reported by many authors that

Table 2. Mortality and Morbidity Rates in 853 Patients Who Underwent Isolated Myocardial Revascularization with Internal Mammary Artery (IMA) Grafts, from April 1991 To April 1992 at the Montreal Heart Institute

	Single IMA	Double IMA	p Value
No. of patients	453	400	
Age (years)	64 ± 0.4	58 ± 0.5	0.00001
Sex (M/F)	321/132	354/46	0.00001
Mean no. of saphenous vein grafts/patient	1.6 ± 0.1	1 ± 0.1	0.00001
Early deaths	7 (1.5%)	9 (2.3%)	0.45
Cardiac complications			
Arrhythmias	73 (16.1%)	57 (14.3%)	0.45
Myocardial infarction	10 (2.2%)	8 (2.0%)	0.83
Heart failure	4 (0.9%)	3 (0.8%)	0.83
Noncardiac complications			
Pleuropulmonary	29 (6.4%)	52 (13.0%)	0.001
Hemorrhage	14 (3.0%)	10 (2.5%)	0.60
Wound infection	4 (0.9%)	8 (2.0%)	0.17
Sternal dehiscence	2 (0.4%)	3 (0.8%)	0.56
Psychiatric	4 (0.9%)	3 (0.8%)	0.83
Neurologic	3 (0.7%)	4 (1.0%)	0.59
Other infections	7 (1.5%)	4 (1.0%)	0.48
Vascular	2 (0.4%)	1 (0.3%)	0.64
Renal	2 (0.4%)	4 (1.0%)	0.33
Gastrointestinal	4 (0.9%)	0	0.06

bilateral IMA grafts improve clinical results of coronary bypass surgery in selected patients (Table 3).[25-30] The incidence of myocardial infarction and of recurrent angina pectoris was significantly lower after double mammary grafting. From these clinical experiences, it appears that the use of bilateral internal mammary artery grafting may decrease late recurrence of cardiac events, but its effect on patient survival remains unclear.

A source of concern after bilateral IMA grafting is the reported higher rate of sternal wound infection.[31,32] Kouchoukos and collaborators[33] found an incidence of 6.9% after double mammary grafting compared to 1.9% after unilateral mammary grafting. They concluded that obesity, diabetes and pulmonary complications were significant risk factors for sternal wound infection. Our own recent experience indicates an incidence of wound infection after double mammary grafting of only 2%, which may result from our more selective approach. We consider morbid obesity, insulin-dependent diabetes mellitus, severe chronic pulmonary disease, and advanced age as

Table 3. Late Survival and Angiographic Results after Bilateral Internal Mammary Artery Grafting

Authors	Year of Report	No. of Patients	Patency Rates (no. of grafts studied)		Mean Time of Study (years)	Patient Survival 10 years	15 years
			LIMA	RIMA			
Barner[29]	1974	100	97% (84)	95% (84)	0.1		
Lytle et al[30]	1983	76	93% (28)	93% (14)	2	90%*	
Galbut et al[22]	1990	1045	92% (63)	85% (53)	4.4	80%	60%
Fiore et al[23]	1990	91	82% (181)	85% (91)	13	84%	74%
Naunheim et al[24]	1992	94				76%	63%

LIMA: left internal mammary artery graft
RIMA: right internal mammary artery graft
* At 9 years of follow-up

contraindications to the use of bilateral mammary artery grafts. Reoperation for coronary artery bypass is not a contraindication, and Galbut and coworkers[34] have reported excellent immediate and long-term results after bilateral internal mammary artery grafting in those patients.[35]

Bilateral and sequential IMA grafting have been advocated by some authors (Table 4).[36-47] Excellent early results have been reported by the group of Dion[42] with the use of sequential mammary grafting in 231 consecutive patients. Technical difficulties did not increase the perioperative mortality and morbidity, and their early graft patency was excellent but no long-term

Table 4. Angiographic Evaluation of Sequential Internal Mammary Artery Grafting

Authors	Year of Report	No. of Patients	No. of Sequential Anastomoses Studied	Early Patency Rate
McBride and Barner[36]	1983	39	20	100%
Kamath et al[37]	1985	87	84	93%
Russo et al[38]	1986	45	108	98%
Tector et al[39]	1986	100	27	93%
Rankin et al[40]	1986	207	155	99%
Jones et al[41]	1987	114	83	96%
Dion et al[42]	1989	231	342	95%
van Sterkenburg[43]	1992	116	229	96%

evaluation of this approach is yet available. With the excellent early clinical and angiographic results, these authors recommended this approach in young, well-selected, low-risk patients. Throughout 1991, bilateral internal mammary artery grafting with sequential anastomoses was performed in only 14 patients of our series (4%). This approach was chosen for selected patients with perfect anatomic conditions, because of the technical difficulty and risk of distal occlusion of the mammary grafts.

In order to expand the use of IMA grafts, Loop and colleagues[48] recommended to use the IMA as a free graft or aortocoronary mammary graft and they reported excellent early and late results. One hundred sixty-six free aortocoronary mammary grafts were performed in 156 patients. The 10-year survival was 77%, and 91% of the 35 grafts studied angiographically after an average of 94 months of follow-up were patent. Landymore and Chapman[49] have shown that the vasa vasorum of the IMA were restrained to the adventitia and did not penetrate the medial layer of the artery. This observation suggests that the IMA wall is nourished from the arterial lumen, and that the artery can be harvested as a free graft without causing ischemic injury to the arterial wall.

The internal mammary artery graft has also been used with excellent early results in patients older than 70 years,[50,51] in children with severe Kawasaki heart disease,[52,53] in patients with smaller body size,[54] in patients on long-term renal dialysis,[55] and in patients with familial hypercholesterolemia.[56] The good results obtained in these various and difficult clinical conditions confirm the versatility of IMA grafting.

EARLY AND LATE GRAFT PATENCY

The early and late patency of left IMA graft to the anterior descending coronary artery has been extensively studied (Tables 1,3). Late patency is better with IMA than with saphenous vein grafts. On the contrary, patency of the right IMA has been shown by some to be underoptimal. Huddleston and collaborators[57] found that the patency of right IMA is similar to that of saphenous vein grafts at 10 years. Loop and his group[58] recommend the use of the right IMA as a free graft rather than as an in situ graft in order to avoid crossing of the midline anteriorly or through the transverse sinus route to the circumflex coronary artery. Free grafts are more versatile to reach the distal branches of the circumflex artery. In addition, the late patency rate of the right mammary graft channeled through the transverse sinus has been the object of concern.[40] Kirklin's group[19] do not recommend its use for grafting the right or the circumflex coronary arteries because of the controversial results reported.

***Table 5. Angiographic Evaluation of Double Internal Mammary Artery
Grafts in 83 Patients Operated Upon at the Montreal Heart Institute
Between 1984 and 1992***

Conduit	Bypassed Coronary Artery	No. of Grafts	Patency Rate	Patency Without Significant Graft Stenosis
LIMA	LAD	52	92%	87%
	Circumflex	25	100%	88%
RIMA	LAD	27	89%	78%
	Circumflex*	25	92%	88%
	Right coronary	17	82%	71%

LAD: left anterior descending artery
LIMA: left internal mammary artery
RIMA: right internal mammary artery
* Through transverse sinus

In our series, 83 patients underwent angiographic evaluation after an average of four months following bilateral mammary artery grafting (Table 5). In 63 patients the angiographic study was obtained to determine patency in the initial experience with the surgical technique. In 20 patients the angiography was done because of recurrence of angina after surgery. The patency rate of left IMA grafts was 90%, that of the right IMA to the left anterior descending coronary artery was 89%, and 92% of right IMA grafts to the circumflex artery through the transverse sinus were patent (Figure 2). These results contrast with the report by Rankin and colleagues[40] indicating a lower patency rate for right IMA grafts through the transverse sinus. In our experience, the lowest patency rate (82%) was found with the use of the right IMA to the right coronary artery.

Nineteen patients with bilateral and sequential IMA grafting underwent angiographic evaluation an average of two months after surgery (Table 6). The patency rate of 42 sequential anastomoses was 86%. Among the six occluded anastomoses, three were distal anastomoses at the anterior descending coronary artery. Dion and collaborators[42] reported a patency rate of 94% in 342 sequential internal mammary artery anastomoses, with a significantly lower patency rate for distal anastomoses than for proximal laterolateral anastomoses. Van Sterkenburg and his group[43] found that 4 of 67 distal anastomoses of sequential left IMA grafts were occluded within one month of surgery. Morin and his colleagues,[59] using the two terminal branches of the internal mammary artery in a Y configuration to graft two major coronary vessels, have obtained the very low early patency rate of 58% among 60 anastomoses studied.

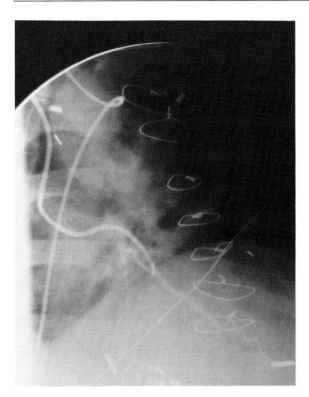

Figure 2. Angiogram of a normal right internal mammary artery graft channeled through the transverse sinus to a circumflex artery.

They concluded that the use of the IMA as a Y graft was technically feasible, but that the early graft patency was dismal, at least during the initial experience.

Overall, while the early IMA patency rate is similar to that of vein grafts, the long-term patency is significantly better, thanks to the absence of atherosclerotic graft disease in IMA grafts. Our experience with the right internal mammary artery to the circumflex coronary artery through the transverse sinus has been favorable. The distal anastomosis to the anterior descending coronary artery is at risk when a sequential graft is performed, and caution in the use of this approach is advised.

Table 6. Angiographic Evaluation of Double and Sequential Internal Mammary Artery Grafts in 19 Patients Who Underwent Operation at the Montreal Heart Institute Between 1984 and 1992

Total number of mammary-coronary anastomoses:	62
Total number of sequential mammary-coronary anastomoses:	42
Patency rate without significant stenosis of sequential grafts:	86%

SPECIFIC COMPLICATIONS WITH THE USE OF IMA GRAFTS

Sternal Wound Complications

IMA grafting and particularly bilateral grafts have been related to a higher incidence of sternal wound dehiscence and infection.[60] On the other hand, Loop and his group[61] found that bilateral IMA grafts in nondiabetic patients carried no greater risk of wound complications.[61] In a recent study of sternal bone healing by tomoscintigraphy performed seven days and one month after surgery, it was shown that IMA dissection causes a significant but temporary devascularization of the sternal bone.[62] The devascularized bone area was greater after bilateral IMA dissection, averaging $24 \pm 6\%$ of total sternal bone, compared to $13 \pm 3\%$ following unilateral IMA dissection, seven days after operation (Figure 3). At one month, the sternal vascularization was normalized in both groups. Therefore, IMA dissection causes a significant although transient devascularization of the sternal bone, which may be responsible for the higher incidence of wound complications reported with IMA grafting.[63-65]

Treatment of sternal wound complications must be aggressive, with early surgical debridement, omental transfer, or mobilization of pectoralis muscle flaps to control and limit the infectious process and accelerate wound closure.[66-69] Between 1982 and 1988, 24 of our patients with sternal wound

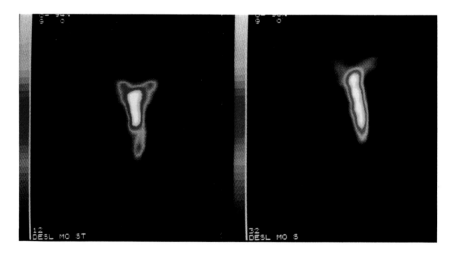

Figure 3. Sternal scintitomogram obtained one week after bilateral internal mammary dissection. There is no or minimal uptake of the radioactive tracer by the distal half of the sternum. The area of hypoperfusion involves 39% of the total sternal area (left). Follow-up study one month after operation (right). There is a diffuse and homogeneous uptake in the sternum (yellow color). No area of hypoactivity is seen.

Table 7. Results of Percutaneous Angioplasty of Internal Mammary Artery Graft Stenoses

Authors	Year of Report	No. of Dilated Grafts	Early Success Rate
Douglas et al[74]	1983	1	0
Zaidi and Hollman[75]	1985	1	100%
Kereiakes et al[76]	1985	2	100%
Côté et al[77]	1987	5	100%
Pinkerton et al[78]	1988	13	92%
Shimshak et al[79]	1988	32	94%
Webb et al[80]	1990	18	67%
Montreal Heart Institute	Unpublished data	22	77%

infection were treated with pectoralis muscle flaps and five others with omental transfer.[70] Four of the patients with pectoralis muscle transfer eventually died of sepsis, whereas all five patients treated with omental transfer recovered uneventfully.

GRAFT VASOSPASM

Vasospasm of IMA grafts due to dissection and surgical handling may sometimes cause life-threatening hemodynamic instability.[71] The use of intraluminal and topical papaverine infusion during surgical preparation of IMA may prevent at least partly this problem.[72,73] During the postoperative period, continuous infusion of nitroglycerin and administration of calcium channel blockers have decreased the incidence of IMA spasm significantly in our experience.

STENOSIS OF THE IMA GRAFT

Early stenosis of the IMA grafts is a rare complication and appears to be more frequent at the distal mammary-coronary anastomosis. Surgical trauma to the coronary or to the internal mammary artery at the anastomotic site and the resulting intimal hyperplasia, or snaring effect of the suture line may be involved. IMA graft angiography should be performed early when angina recurs after operation to eliminate the possibility of an anastomotic stenosis.

Between 1983 and 1992 a significant mammary graft stenosis was found in 20 patients evaluated angiographically for recurrence of angina following

IMA grafting. Sixteen stenoses were at a left IMA to anterior descending coronary artery anastomosis, one at the anastomosis of the left IMA to the first marginal circumflex artery, one at a right mammary to right coronary artery anastomosis, one at a right mammary to anterior descending coronary artery, and two at right IMA to left marginal circumflex anastomoses. Only one stenosis was found at the origin of a right mammary artery grafted to the circumflex coronary artery. The average interval between initial operation and diagnosis of IMA stenosis was just over two years. Percutaneous angioplasty of the mammary artery graft or of the mammary to coronary anastomosis was performed on 22 grafts, with an early success rate of 77%, an experience similar to that of others (Table 7).[74-80] Late results are not yet clearly established, although there are indications that the recurrence rate may be lowest for stenoses of the distal anastomosis.[81]

STENOSIS OF THE SUBCLAVIAN ARTERY

Blood flow in IMA grafts may be impaired by a stenosis of the subclavian artery with resulting myocardial ischemia. A subclavian artery stenosis was found in four of our patients before internal mammary artery grafting, and

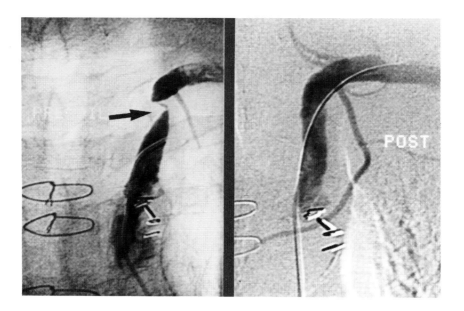

Figure 4. Angiogram of a left subclavian artery stenosis (left, arrow). After percutaneous transluminal angioplasty, the stenosis is completely relieved (right).

in six patients after coronary bypass grafting with in situ internal mammary artery grafts. Percutaneous transluminal angioplasty of the subclavian artery was successfully performed in the four patients with the preoperative finding and in five of the six patients with recurring angina after IMA grafting (Figure 4). No evidence of restenosis was found at continuous wave Doppler study, an average of 38 months after dilatation, and nine patients remained free of angina. One patient developed complete occlusion of the subclavian artery, and a carotid-subclavian bypass was performed because of recurrence of angina.

The incidence of atherosclerosis in the subclavian artery ranges from 0.5 to 2% in angiographic and clinical series.[82,83] Doppler flow study is indicated before IMA grafting whenever there are clinical signs of subclavian artery stenosis, or when angina recurs following IMA grafting. Laub and coworkers[84] have recommended to avoid the use of IMA in the presence of subclavian artery stenosis, or to use it as a free graft. However in selected patients, preoperative dilatation of the subclavian artery may be a useful alternative, although long-term results are still uncertain. Surgical treatment has been recommended for the treatment of subclavian artery stenosis associated with an IMA graft.[85-88] However, in our hands, percutaneous angioplasty of the subclavian artery has been a safe and effective approach to this problem and myocardial ischemia has been successfully relieved.

TECHNICAL ASPECTS OF IMA GRAFTING

IN SITU IMA GRAFTS

The many surgical considerations and technical aspects of IMA grafting have been well described.[89] Only the most important technical factors that in our opinion may have a bearing on the success rate of IMA grafts will be emphasized here.

IMA grafts are prepared by harvesting a 1 cm large pedicle of endothoracic fascia and muscle; the is dissection performed using the electrocautery at a low energy level (20 watts). The artery is freed from the chest wall down to below its bifurcation into the musculophrenic artery and the superior epigastric artery distally. Proximally, the dissection is carried up to the subclavian artery, being careful to avoid injury to the phrenic nerve which lies medially and posteriorly to the origin of the mammary artery. The right internal mammary artery may be constrained proximally by lateral pleural attachments. Cutting of pleural attachments and adhesions and dividing the right mammary vein provides additional length to the right IMA.[90] The IMA pedicles are sprayed with a papaverine solution, and cut distally at the beginning of cardiopulmonary bypass, or immediately before performing the anastomosis. Contrary to others,[91] we do not use intraluminal injection of papaverine routinely, but only when free mammary artery flow appears inadequate. Minimal manipulation and trauma to the mammary artery are mandatory to protect the endothelial cell function.[92,93]

The mammary to coronary anastomosis with a 8-0 monofilament continuous suture is performed under optical magnification. To prevent traction and angulation, the mammary pedicle is fixed to the epicardium, after all distal anastomoses are completed. The pericardium is left widely open and incisions are made to avoid kinking of the mammary graft with lung inflation.[94] A pericardial flap is sutured to the chest wall to prevent traction on the left IMA by the inflated left lung.[95-97] Buxton and Knight[98] and Pacificio and colleagues[99] have proposed to channel the IMA through the pericardium behind the phrenic nerve, a technique which is rarely necessary.

Table 8. Mortality and Morbidity Rates in 39 Patients Who Underwent Combined Valve Replacement and Internal Mammary Artery Grafting in 1991 and 1992 at the Montreal Heart Institute

Age (years)	66 ± 1	
Sex (M/F)	23 / 16	
Mean no. IMA grafts/patient	1	
Mean no. SV grafts/patient	1 ± 0.1	
AVR (no.)	27	
MVR (no.)	11	
Double valve replacement (no.)	1	
Mechanical prosthesis (no.)	22	
Bioprosthesis (no.)	18	
Hospital death (no.)	4	(10%)
Complications (no.)		
Arrhythmias	6	(15%)
Myocardial infarction	1	(3%)
Pleuropulmonary	6	(15%)
Hemorrhage	5	(13%)
Wound infection	2	(5%)
Neurologic	1	(3%)

AVR: aortic valve replacement
IMA: internal mammary artery
MVR: mitral valve replacement
SV: saphenous vein

Most often the left IMA is used for grafting of the anterior descending coronary artery, but it can also serve to bypass the circumflex territory. The right IMA can be used as a graft to the right, the anterior descending, or the first marginal circumflex arteries. In the latter case, it has to be channeled through the transverse sinus, as described by Puig and his group.[100]

When the left IMA is anastomosed to the anterior descending coronary artery, the right IMA serves to graft the next largest coronary territory.[101,102] Additional grafts are most often needed to achieve complete myocardial revascularization.[103] The choice is then between saphenous vein grafts, the gastroepiploic artery, the inferior epigastric artery or sequential IMA grafts. In our experience saphenous vein grafts were most often used in association with IMA grafts (Table 2). Sequential IMA grafting and alternative arterial conduits were used only in well-selected patients.

SEQUENTIAL MAMMARY ARTERY GRAFTING

Several important technical considerations in the performance of complex IMA grafting procedures have been described by many, stressing the pitfalls and dangers of using the IMA as a sequential graft.[41-46,104,105] Under optimal anatomic conditions and with an IMA of suitable size and length, a sequential IMA graft can be constructed to the anterior descending coronary artery and to a major diagonal branch. It is rarely indicated to use a sequential IMA graft to other coronary arteries.

FREE IMA GRAFTS

With free IMA grafts, the use of this arterial conduit may be widened. Whenever it appears that a mammary graft is too short, before, during or after completion of the coronary anastomosis, the proximal end of the IMA can be ligated and severed to be implanted on the ascending aorta with a 7-0 monofilament continuous suture. When the aorta is thick or diseased, it may be useful to construct the proximal anastomosis on the hood of a vein graft, or on a vein patch graft sutured to the aortic wall.[48]

IMA GRAFT AND VALVE REPLACEMENT

In 1991 and 1992, the left IMA was used for coronary bypass in 39 patients undergoing valve replacement (Table 8). Both mechanical and biological valves were used, and the left IMA served to bypass the anterior descending coronary artery in all these patients. The hospital mortality was 10%, and no death was related to coronary grafting. Our results are similar

Table 9. Clinical and Angiographic Characteristics of 82 Patients with Unstable Angina and Previous Coronary Artery Bypass Grafting. Experience of the Montreal Heart Institute from 1990 to 1992

	Patients with Vein Grafts (n = 59)		Patients with IMA Grafts (n = 23)		p Value
Age (years)	62 ± 1		59 ± 2		0.15
Sex (M/F)	55/4		22/1		0.68
Mean interval* (months)	108 ± 6		48 ± 6		0.01
Native coronary angiography (no. with stenosis > 50%)					
Left main	17/54	(31%)	5/20	(25%)	0.58
LAD	47/54	(87%)	19/20	(95%)	0.33
Circumflex	42/54	(78%)	17/20	(85%)	0.49
Right coronary	51/54	(94%)	18/20	(90%)	0.50
Vein grafts with stenosis > 50%					
to LAD artery	18/36	(50%)	0/1		
to circumflex artery	28/33	(85%)	6/11	(55%)	0.04
to right coronary artery	16/30	(53%)	9/13	(69%)	0.33
Patent IMA grafts (no.)			21/23	(91%)	
Left ventricle ejection fraction (%)	58 ± 2		58 ± 3		0.94
Hospital complications					
Refractory angina	11	(19%)	2	(9%)	0.27
Myocardial infarction	12	(20%)	2	(9%)	0.21
Death	2	(3%)	0		0.37
Medical treatment only	32	(54%)	15	(65%)	0.37
Angioplasty	12	(20%)	8	(35%)	0.17
Reoperation	15	(25%)	0		0.01

IMA: internal mammary artery
LAD: left anterior descending coronary artery
* Mean interval between coronary artery bypass surgery and episode of unstable angina

to those reported with combined valve replacement and saphenous vein grafting.[106-108]

In this experience we have seen no evidence that the IMA was inadequate to meet the need in blood flow of the hypertrophied left ventricle. Therefore, in selected young patients, in cases of severely diseased ascending aorta, and in the absence of suitable vein grafts, an IMA graft can be safely used to bypass the anterior descending or marginal coronary arteries, without increasing surgical mortality and morbidity.

IMA GRAFTS AT REOPERATION

Reoperation for coronary artery bypass grafting is a technical challenge which is even more difficult in the presence of a previous IMA graft.[109] Baillot and coauthors[110] reported on a series of 100 consecutive patients with a patent IMA graft who underwent coronary artery reoperation. Occlusion of saphenous vein grafts and progression of disease in ungrafted coronary arteries were the indications for reoperation. Eight IMA pedicles were damaged at reoperation and the operative mortality was 1%. According to Coltharp and his group,[111] early complication and mortality rates of reoperation do not differ significantly between patients with and those without prior IMA grafting.

UNSTABLE ANGINA IN PATIENTS WITH PREVIOUS IMA GRAFTING

Previous coronary bypass grafting with saphenous vein grafts is an adverse prognosis factor in unstable angina.[112] Twenty-one percent of the patients admitted with unstable angina at the Montreal Heart Institute in recent years have had previous coronary artery bypass surgery.[113] This has become a significant problem following coronary surgery and it is expected to grow as the number of patients with previous surgery and the interval since the operation increase.

Between December 1990 and March 1992, 82 patients with previous coronary bypass surgery were admitted to the hospital for unstable angina (Table 9). Fifty-nine of the patients had saphenous vein grafts only, and 23 patients had at least one IMA graft. Age, sex and the anatomy of native coronary artery disease were similar in both groups. The interval between initial operation and the episode of unstable angina was significantly shorter in the group with IMA grafts. The incidence of hospital complications was lower among patients with an IMA graft than in those with saphenous vein grafts, but the difference was not statistically significant. Whereas all patients with an IMA graft were controlled with medical treatment[114] and angioplasty, 25% of the patients with saphenous vein grafts required reoperation for coronary artery bypass.

Long-term follow-up of these patients will determine the effect of IMA grafts on recurrence of cardiac events, but on the short-term, nonoperative treatment was successful to control angina in all patients with previous IMA grafts, contrary to those with vein grafts only.

EFFECT OF IMA GRAFTING ON SUBSEQUENT HOSPITALIZATIONS

Following coronary artery bypass grafting with saphenous vein grafts the rate of subsequent hospitalizations is significantly less than that among patients with similar coronary disease treated medically.[115] Loop and coworkers[7] have found that IMA grafting to the left anterior descending coronary artery decreases the risk of late myocardial infarction, that of subsequent hospitalizations, and of postoperative cardiac events, when compared to

Table 10. Influence of Internal Mammary Artery Grafting on Subsequent Rehospitalization from 1985 to 1991 at the Montreal Heart Institute

	Single IMA Grafting	Double IMA Grafting	p Value
Number of patients	2775	1741	
Number of early rehospitalization (< 1 year)	227 (8%)	140 (8%)	0.87
Number of late rehospitalization (> 1 year)	249 (9%)	103 (6%)	0.0002
Total	476 (17%)	243 (14%)	0.004

patients with saphenous vein grafts. In a preliminary analysis of the Medicare data base, Roper and collaborators[116] found that the readmission rate of patients was lower following coronary artery bypass surgery than after percutaneous transluminal coronary angioplasty.

Among the patients followed at the Montreal Heart Institute, between 1985 and 1991, 8% of those with IMA grafts were rehospitalized during the first year following surgery (Table 10). Postoperative surgical complications were the main cause for rehospitalization. Nine percent of the patients with single IMA were rehospitalized during late follow-up, compared to 6% of those with double IMA grafts (p < 0.05). Late rehospitalization in both groups was mainly due to recurrence of angina.

A decrease in late cardiac events and in reoperation rate among patients with bilateral IMA grafts was also reported by Fiore's group.[23] Data are accumulating in support of the hypothesis that double IMA grafting improves the late outcome of patients undergoing myocardial revascularization. The issue of quality of care for patients with coronary artery disease is not negligible in the present era of efficiency analysis and cost containment. Despite the absence of a consensus on the advantages of bilateral IMA grafting on survival, current data on long-term cardiac events and rehospitalization rate following surgery strongly favor the use of bilateral IMA grafting, whenever it is clinically indicated and technically feasible.

CONCLUSION

The quest for the optimal conduit for coronary artery bypass grafting is led by clinical outcome and long-term patency, the former being dependent upon the latter. Current experience indicates that IMA grafts can achieve this goal better than vein grafts, mainly because they remain free from accelerated atherosclerotic graft disease, resulting in fewer further cardiac events and rehospitalization, and in prolonged survival of the patients. Whether or not other arterial grafts such as the right gastroepiploic and the inferior epigastric arteries will also contribute to improve the late outcome of myocardial revascularization remains to be determined. Needless to say that secondary prevention with proper dieting and lipid-lowering pharmacologic treatment is also necessary to decrease the progression of disease in native coronary vessels and to prevent recurrence of myocardial ischemia.

REFERENCES

1. Grondin CM, Campeau L, Lespérance J et al. Comparison of late changes in internal mammary artery and saphenous vein grafts in two consecutive series of patients 10 years after operation. Circulation 1984; 70(suppl):I-208-I-2.

2. Singh RN, Sosa JA, Green GE. Long-term fate of the internal mammary artery and saphenous vein grafts. J Thorac Cardiovasc Surg 1983; 86:359-63.

3. Loop FD, Irarrazaval MJ, Bredee JJ et al. Internal mammary artery graft for ischemic heart disease. Effect of revascularization on clinical status and survival. Am J Cardiol 1977; 39:516-22.

4. Tector AJ, Schmahl TM, Janon B et al. The internal mammary artery graft. Its longevity after coronary bypass. JAMA 1981; 246:2181-3.

5. Tector AJ, Schmahl TM, Canino VR. The internal mammary artery graft: The best choice for bypass of the diseased left anterior descending coronary artery. Circulation 1983; 68(suppl):II-214-II-7.

6. Acinapura AJ, Rose DM, Jacobowitz IJ et al. Internal mammary artery bypass grafting: Influence on recurrent angina and survival in 2100 patients. Ann Thorac Surg 1989; 48:186-91.

7. Loop FD, Lytle BW, Cosgrove DM et al. Influence of the internal mammary artery graft on 10-year survival and other cardiac events. N Engl J Med 1986; 314:1-6.

8. Okies JE, Page SU, Bigelow JC et al. The left internal mammary artery: The graft of choice. Circulation 1984; 70(suppl):I-213-I-21.

9. Barner HB, Standeven JW, Reese J. Twelve year experience with internal mammary artery for coronary artery bypass. J Thorac Cardiovasc Surg 1985; 90:668-75.

10. Olearchyk AS, Magovern GJ. Internal mammary artery grafting: Clinical results, patency rates, and long-term survival in 833 patients. J Thorac Cardiovasc Surg 1986; 92:1082-7.

11. Cameron A, Kemp HG, Green GE. Bypass surgery with the internal mammary artery graft: 15 years follow-up. Circulation 1986; 74(suppl):III-30-III-6.

12. Ivert T, Huttunen K, Landou C et al. Angiographic studies of internal mammary artery grafts 11 years after coronary artery bypass grafting. J Thorac Cardiovasc Surg 1988; 96:1-12.

13. Zeff RH, Kongtahworn C, Iannone LA et al. Internal mammary artery versus saphenous vein graft to the left anterior descending coronary artery: Prospective randomized study with 10-year follow-up. Ann Thorac Surg 1988; 45:533-6.

14. Kirklin JW, Naftel DC, Blackstone EH et al. Summary of a consensus concerning death and ischemic events after coronary artery bypass grafting. Circulation 1989; 79(suppl):I-81-I-91.

15. Johnson WD, Brenowitz JB, Kayser KL. Factors influencing long-term (10-years to 15-years) survival after a successful coronary artery bypass operation. Ann Thorac Surg 1989; 48:19-25.

16. Cosgrove DM, Loop FD, Lytle BW et al. Predictors of reoperation after myocardial revascularization. J Thorac Cardiovasc Surg 1986; 92:811-21.

17. Killen DA, Arnold MA, McConahay DR. Fifteen-year results of coronary artery bypass for isolated left anterior descending coronary artery disease. Ann Thorac Surg 1989; 47:595-9.

18. Cameron A, Davis KB, Green GE et al. Clinical implications of internal mammary artery bypass grafts: The coronary artery surgery study experience. Circulation 1988; 77:815-9.

19. Kirklin JW, Akins CW, Blackstone EH et al. Guidelines and indications for coronary artery bypass graft surgery. J Am Coll Cardiol 1991; 17:543-89.

20. Frye RL, Gibbons RJ, Schaff HV et al. Treatment of coronary artery disease. J Am Coll Cardiol 1989; 13:957-68.

21. Richenbacher WE, Myers JL, Waldhausen JA. Current status of cardiac surgery: A 40-year review. J Am Coll Cardiol 1989; 14:535-44.

22. Galbut DL, Traad EA, Dorman MJ et al. Seventeen-year experience with bilateral internal mammary artery grafts. Ann Thorac Surg 1990; 49:195-201.

23. Fiore AC, Naunheim KS, Dean P et al. Results of internal thoracic artery grafting over 15 years: Single versus double grafts. Ann Thorac Surg 1990; 49:202-9.

24. Naunheim KS, Barner HB, Fiore AC. Update. Ann Thorac Surg 1992; 53:716-8.

25. Galbut DL, Traad EA, Dorman MJ et al. Twelve-year experience with bilateral internal mammary artery grafts. Ann Thorac Surg 1985; 40:264-70.

26. Finci L, von Segesser L, Meier B et al. Comparison of multivessel coronary angioplasty with surgical revascularization with both internal mammary arteries. Circulation 1987; 76(suppl):V-1-V-5.

27. Jones EL, Lutz JF, King SB et al. Extended use of the internal mammary artery graft: Important anatomic and physiologic considerations. Circulation 1986; 74(suppl):III-41-III-7.

28. Henze A, Ramström J, Nyström SO. Bilateral internal mammary artery for coronary revascularization. Scand J Thorac Cardiovasc Surg 1989; 23:9-12.

29. Barner HB. Double internal mammary coronary artery bypass. Arch Surg 1974; 109:627-30.

30. Lytle BW, Cosgrove DM, Saltus GL et al. Multivessel coronary revascularization without saphenous vein: Long-term results of bilateral internal mammary artery grafting. Ann Thorac Surg 1983; 36:540-7.

31. Cosgrove DM, Lytle BW, Loop FD et al. Does bilateral internal mammary artery grafting increase surgical risk? J Thorac Cardiovasc Surg 1988; 95:850-6.

32. Lytle BW, Cosgrove DM, Loop FD et al. Perioperative risk of bilateral internal mammary artery grafting: Analysis of 500 cases from 1971 to 1984. Circulation 1986; 74(suppl):III-37-III-41.

33. Kouchoukos NT, Wareing TH, Murphy SF et al. Risks of bilateral internal mammary artery bypass grafting. Ann Thorac Surg 1990; 49:210-9.

34. Galbut DL, Traad EA, Dorman MJ et al. Bilateral internal mammary artery grafts in reoperative and primary coronary bypass surgery. Ann Thorac Surg 1991; 52:20-8.

35. Loop FD, Lytle BW, Cosgrove DM. Bilateral internal thoracic artery grafting in reoperations. Ann Thorac Surg 1991; 52:3-4.

36. McBride LR, Barner HB. The left internal mammary artery as a sequential graft to the left anterior descending system. J Thorac Cardiovasc Surg 1983; 86:703-5.

37. Kamath ML, Matyski LS, Schmidt DH et al. Sequential internal mammary artery grafts. J Thorac Cardiovasc Surg 1985; 89:163-9.

38. Russo P, Orzulak TA, Schaff H et al. Use of internal mammary artery grafts for multiple coronary artery bypass. Circulation 1986; 74(suppl):III-48-III-52.

39. Tector AJ, Schmahl TM, Canino VR. Expanding the use of the internal mammary artery to improve patency in coronary artery bypass grafting. J Thorac Cardiovasc Surg 1986; 91:9-16.

40. Rankin JS, Newman GE, Bashore TM et al. Clinical and angiographic assessment of complex thoracic artery bypass grafting. J Thorac Cardiovasc Surg 1986; 92:832-46.

41. Jones EL, Lattouf O, Lutz JF et al. Important anatomic and physiologic considerations in performance of complex mammary-coronary artery operations. Ann Thorac Surg 1987; 43:469-77.

42. Dion R, Verhelst R, Rousseau M et al. Sequential mammary grafting. J Thorac Cardiovasc Surg 1989; 98:80-9.

43. van Sterkenburg SM, Ernst SMPG, de la Riviere AB et al. Triple sequential grafts using the internal mammary artery. J Thorac Cardiovasc Surg 1992; 104:60-5.

44. Kabbani SS, Hanna ES, Bashour TT et al. Sequential internal mammary coronary artery bypass. J Thorac Cardiovasc Surg 1983; 86:697-702.

45. Tector A, Schmahl TM, Canino VR et al. The role of the sequential mammary artery graft in coronary surgery. Circulation 1984; 70(suppl):I-222-I-5.

46. Boustany CW, Mills NL. Sequential coronary artery bypass utilizing the internal mammary artery. J Cardiovasc Surg 1988; 29:123-7.

47. Sergeant P, Flameng W, Suy R. The sequential internal mammary artery graft. J Cardiovasc Surg 1988; 29:596-600.

48. Loop FD, Lytle BW, Cosgrove DM et al. Free aortocoronary internal mammary artery graft: Late results. J Thorac Cardiovasc Surg 1986; 92:827-31.

49. Landymore RW, Chapman DM. Anatomical studies to support the expanded use of the internal mammary artery graft for myocardial revascularization. Ann Thorac Surg 1987; 44:4-6.

50. Azariades M, Fessler CL, Floten HS et al. Five-year results of coronary bypass grafting for patients older than 70 years: Role of internal mammary artery. Ann Thorac Surg 1990; 50:940-5.

51. Gardner TJ, Greene PS, Rykiel MF et al. Routine use of the left internal mammary artery graft in the elderly. Ann Thorac Surg 1990; 49:188-94.

52. Kitamura S, Kawachi K, Oyama C et al. Severe Kawasaki heart disease treated with an internal mammary artery graft in pediatric patients. J Thorac Cardiovasc Surg 1985; 89:860-6.

53. Kitamura S, Kawachi K, Seki T et al. Bilateral internal mammary artery grafts for coronary artery bypass operations in children. J Thorac Cardiovasc Surg 1990; 99:708-15.

54. Suma H, Takeuchi A, Kondo K et al. Internal mammary artery grafting in patients with smaller body structure. J Thorac Cardiovasc Surg 1988; 96:393-9.

55. Blakeman B, Sullivan HJ, Foy BK et al. Internal mammary artery revascularization in the patient on long-term renal dialysis. Ann Thorac Surg 1990; 50:776-8.

56. Reeves F, Gosselin G, Hébert Y et al. Long-term follow-up after portacaval shunt and internal mammary coronary bypass graft in homozygous familial hypercholesterolemia: Report of two cases. Can J Cardiol 1990; 6:171-4.

57. Huddleston CB, Stoney WS, Alford WC et al. Internal mammary artery grafts: Technical factors influencing patency. Ann Thorac Surg 1986; 42:543-9.

58. Loop FD, Lytle BW, Cosgrove DM. Bilateral internal mammary artery grafting in reoperations. Ann Thorac Surg 1991; 52:3-4.

59. Morin JE, Hedderich G, Poirier NL et al. Coronary artery bypass using internal mammary artery branches. Ann Thorac Surg 1992; 54:911-4.

60. Grossi EA, Esposito R, Crooke GA et al. Sternal wound infections and use of internal mammary artery grafts. J Thorac Cardiovasc Surg 1991; 102:342-7.

61. Loop FD, Lytle BW, Cosgrove DM et al. Sternal wound complications after isolated coronary artery bypass grafting: Early and late mortality, morbidity, and cost of care. Ann Thorac Surg 1990; 49:179-87.

62. Carrier M, Grégoire J, Tronc F et al. Effect of internal mammary artery dissection on sternal vascularization. Ann Thorac Surg 1992; 53:115-9.

63. Arnold M. The surgical anatomy of sternal blood supply. Ann Thorac Surg 1972; 64:596-610.

64. Seyfer AE, Shriver CD, Miller TR et al. Sternal blood flow after median sternotomy and mobilization of the internal mammary arteries. Surgery 1988; 104:899-904.

65. Grmoljez PF, Barner HB. Bilateral internal mammary artery mobilization and sternal healing. Angiology 1978; 29:272-4.

66. Scully H, Leclerc Y, Martin R et al. Comparison between antibiotic irrigation and mobilization of pectoral muscle flaps in treatment of deep sternal infections. J Thorac Cardiovasc Surg 1985; 90:523-31.

67. Mathisen DJ, Grillo HC, Vlahakes GJ et al. The omentum in the management of complicated cardiothoracic problems. J Thorac Cardiovasc Surg 1988; 95:677-84.

68. Heath BJ, Bagnato VJ. Poststernotomy mediastinitis treated by omental transfer without postoperative irrigation or drainage. J Thorac Cardiovasc Surg 1987; 94:355-60.

69. Bedard JP, Shamji F, Keon WJ. Omental pedicle grafting in the treatment of poststernotomy mediastinitis. Can J Surg 1989; 32:328-30.

70. Semper O, Leclerc Y, Cartier R et al. Médiastinite post-sternotomie: Stratégie de traitement. Ann Chir 1991; 45:770-3.

71. Sarabu MR, McClung JA, Fass A et al. Early postoperative spasm in the left internal mammary artery bypass grafts. Ann Thorac Surg 1987; 44:199-200.

72. Hillier C, Watt PAC, Spyt TJ et al. Contraction and relaxation of human internal mammary artery after intraluminal administration of papaverine. Ann Thorac Surg 1992; 53:1033-7.

73. Cooper GJ, Wilkinson GAL, Angelini GD. Overcoming perioperative spasm of the internal mammary artery: Which is the best vasodilator? J Thorac Cardiovasc Surg 1992; 104:465-8.

74. Douglas JS, Gruentzig AR, King SB et al. Percutaneous transluminal coronary angioplasty in patients with prior coronary bypass surgery. J Am Coll Cardiol 1983; 2:745-54.

75. Zaidi AR, Hollman JL. Percutaneous angioplasty of internal mammary graft stenosis: Case report and discussion. Cathet Cardiovasc Diag 1985; 11:603-8.

76. Kereiakes DJ, George B, Stertzer SH et al. Percutaneous transluminal angioplasty of left internal mammary artery grafts. Am J Cardiol 1985; 55:1215-6.

77. Côté G, Myler RK, Stertzer SH et al. Percutaneous transluminal angioplasty of stenotic coronary artery bypass grafts: 5 years' experience. J Am Coll Cardiol 1987; 9:8-17.

78. Pinkerton CA, Slack JD, Orr CM et al. Percutaneous transluminal angioplasty in patients with prior myocardial revascularization surgery. Am J Cardiol 1988; 61:15G-7G.

79. Shimshak TM, Giorgi LV, Johnson WL et al. Application of percutaneous transluminal coronary angioplasty to the internal mammary artery graft. J Am Coll Cardiol 1988; 12:1205-14.

80. Webb JG, Myler RK, Shaw RE et al. Coronary angioplasty after coronary bypass surgery: Initial results and late outcome in 422 patients. J Am Coll Cardiol 1990; 16:812-20.

81. Waters D, Côté G. Angioplasty of bypass grafts and native arteries. In: Waters DD, Bourassa MG eds. Care of the Patient with Previous Coronary Bypass Surgery. Brest AN, ed. Philadelphia: FA Davis Company, 1991:241-56.

82. Brown AH. Coronary steal by internal mammary graft with subclavian stenosis. J Thorac Cardiovasc Surg 1976; 73:690-3.

83. Shapira S, Braun S, Puram B et al. Percutaneous transluminal angioplasty of proximal subclavian artery after left internal mammary to left anterior descending artery bypass surgery. J Am Coll Cardiol 1991; 18:1120-3.

84. Laub GW, Muralidharan S, Naidech H et al. Percutaneous transluminal subclavian angioplasty in a patient with postoperative angina. Ann Thorac Surg 1991; 52:850-1.

85. Granke K, van Meter CH, White CJ et al. Myocardial ischemia caused by postoperative malfunction of a patent internal mammary arterial graft. J Vasc Surg 1990; 11:659-64.

86. Bashour TT, Crew J, Kabbani SS et al. Symptomatic coronary and cerebral steal after internal mammary coronary bypass. Am Heart J 1984; 108:177-88.

87. Olsen CO, Dunton RF, Maggs PR et al. Review of coronary subclavian steal following internal mammary artery bypass surgery. Ann Thorac Surg 1988; 46:675-8.

88. Tyras DH, Barner HB. Coronary subclavian steal. Arch Surg 1977; 112:1125-7.

89. Jones EL. Preparation of the internal mammary artery for coronary bypass surgery. J Card Surg 1991; 6:326-9.

90. Cosgrove DM, Loop FD. Techniques to maximize mammary artery length. Ann Thorac Surg 1985; 40:78-9.

91. Mills NL, Bringaze W. Preparation of the internal mammary artery graft: Which is the best method? J Thorac Cardiovasc Surg 1989; 98:73-9.

92. Fogarty TJ, Mollenauer KH. Preparation of the internal mammary artery for coronary artery bypass grafting. J Card Surg 1991; 6:322-5.

93. Mills NL. Preparation of the internal mammary artery graft with intraluminal papaverine. J Card Surg 1991; 6:318-21.

94. Van der Salm TJ, Chowdhary S, Okike DN et al. Internal mammary artery grafts: The shortest route to the coronary arteries. Ann Thorac Surg 1989; 47:421-7.

95. Berry BE, Davis DJ, Sheely CH et al. Protection and expanded use or the left internal mammary artery graft by pericardial flap technique. J Thorac Cardiovasc Surg 1988; 95:346-50.

96. Starr DS, Moore JP. Localized pericardial flap to prevent tension on left internal mammary artery grafts. Ann Thorac Surg 1989; 47:623-4.

97. Todd EP, Earle GF, Jaggers R et al. Pericardial flap to minimize internal mammary artery anastomotic tension. Ann Thorac Surg 1987; 44:665-6.

98. Buxton B, Knight S. Retrophrenic location of the internal mammary artery graft. Ann Thorac Surg 1990; 49:1011-2.

99. Pacifico AD, Sears NJ, Bugos C. Harvesting, routing, and anastomosing the left internal mammary artery graft. Ann Thorac Surg 1986; 42:708-10.

100. Puig LB, Neto LF, Rati M et al. A technique of anastomosis of the right internal mammary artery to the circumflex artery and its branch. Ann Thorac Surg 1984; 38:533-46.

101. Geha AS. Crossed double internal mammary to coronary artery grafts: Indications, techniques, and results. Arch Surg 1976; 111:289-92.

102. Sauvage LR, Wu HD, Kowalsky TE et al. Healing basis and surgical technique for complete revascularization of the left ventricle using only the internal mammary arteries. Ann Thorac Surg 1986; 42:449-65.

103. Bell MR, Gersh BJ, Schaff HV et al. Effect of completeness of revascularization on long-term outcome of patients with three-vessel disease undergoing coronary artery bypass surgery. A report from the Coronary Artery Surgery Study (CASS) registry. Circulation 1992; 86:446-57.

104. Jones EL, Lattouf OM, Weintraub WS. Catastrophic consequences of internal mammary artery hypoperfusion. J Thorac Cardiovasc Surg 1989; 98:902-7.

105. Kesler KA, Sharp TG, Turrentine MW et al. Technical considerations and early results of sequential left internal mammary artery bypass grafting to the left anterior descending coronary artery system. J Cardiac Surg 1990; 5:134-44.

106. Johnson WD, Kayser KL, Pedraza P et al. Combined valve replacement and coronary bypass surgery. Chest 1986; 90:338-45.

107. Czer LS, Gray RJ, DeRobertis MA et al. Mitral valve replacement: Impact of coronary artery disease and determinants of prognosis after revascularization. Circulation 1984; 70(suppl):I-198-I-207.

108. Lytle BW, Cosgrove DM, Gill CC et al. Mitral valve replacement combined with myocardial revascularization: Early and late results for 300 patients, 1970 to 1983. Circulation 1985; 71:1179-90.

109. Perrault L, Carrier M, Cartier R et al. Morbidity and mortality of reoperation for coronary artery bypass grafting: Significance of atheromatous vein grafts. Can J Cardiol 1991; 7:427-30.

110. Baillot RG, Loop FD, Cosgrove DM et al. Reoperation after previous grafting with the internal mammary artery: Techniques and early results. Ann Thorac Surg 1985; 40:271-3.

111. Coltharp WH, Decker MD, Lea JW et al. Internal mammary artery graft at reoperation: Risks, benefits, and methods of preservation. Ann Thorac Surg 1991; 52:225-9.

112. Waters DD, Walling A, Roy D et al. Previous coronary artery bypass grafting as an adverse prognosis factor in unstable angina pectoris. Am J Cardiol 1986; 58:465-9.

113. Théroux P, Waters DD. Unstable angina: Special considerations in the post-bypass patient. In: Waters DD, Bourasssa MG, eds. Care of the Patient with Previous Coronary Bypass Surgery. Brest AN, ed. Philadelphia: FA Davis Company, 1991:169-91.

114. Théroux P, Ouimet H, McCans J et al. Aspirin, heparin, or both to treat acute unstable angina. N Engl J Med 1988; 319:1105-11.

115. Hamilton WM, Hammermeister KE, DeRouen TA et al. Effect of coronary artery bypass grafting on subsequent hospitalization. Am J Cardiol 1983; 51:353-60.

116. Roper WL, Winkenwerder W, Hackbarth GM et al. Effectiveness in health care. An initiative to evaluate and improve medical practice. N Engl J Med 1988; 319:1197-202.

CHAPTER 4

NEW ARTERIAL CONDUITS: IS THERE A PLACE FOR THE RIGHT GASTROEPIPLOIC ARTERY AND THE INFERIOR EPIGASTRIC ARTERY?

Louis Perrault
Michel Carrier
L. Conrad Pelletier

INTRODUCTION

The excellent long-term results obtained with the internal mammary artery have stimulated interest for the search of other arterial conduits with similar characteristics that could be useful in achieving complete revascularization with arterial conduits only, thus avoiding the need for vein grafts. In recent years, the right gastroepiploic artery and the inferior epigastric artery have been proposed as adjuvants to internal mammary arteries, and there has been a renewed interest for the radial artery graft.[1]

The use of the right gastroepiploic artery (RGEA) for coronary artery bypass grafting was first proposed by Edwards and his colleagues in 1974,[2] but the interest in this conduit has grown particularly since the report by Pym and his group in 1987.[3] A report by Puig and collaborators in 1988[4] has recently drawn attention toward the inferior epigastric artery (IEA). The experience with these two arterial conduits will be reviewed and their role in coronary artery bypass grafting discussed.

THE RIGHT GASTROEPIPLOIC ARTERY (RGEA) GRAFT

ANATOMY, HISTOLOGY AND PHYSIOLOGY

The RGEA is a branch of the gastroduodenal artery which courses along the greater curvature of the stomach and merges with the left gastroepiploic artery. The length of the RGEA suitable for coronary grafting averages 18 cm. It is therefore most often used to bypass the right coronary artery, although occasionally it may also reach the distal left anterior descending and distal marginal coronary arteries.[5] In most patients, the distal end of the RGEA has an internal diameter of 1 to 1.5 mm and is thus adequate for coronary anastomosis.[5,6] The coeliac and gastroduodenal arteries are rarely infiltrated with atherosclerosis, and the incidence of significant artery stenosis has been reported to be as low as 1%.[7]

Histologically, the RGEA has several similarities with the internal mammary artery in terms of fenestration and of composition of external and internal elastic layers.[6] The RGEA intima is thicker than that of the internal mammary, but significant luminal narrowings are rare.[7] The fact that atherosclerosis develops only to a very mild degree in the RGEA is a strong indication that this vessel has a good long-term potential as a coronary artery bypass graft.

Biochemical studies have shown that the RGEA releases more vasodilatory prostacyclin and endothelium-derived relaxing factors than saphenous vein grafts.[8-11] On the other hand, the RGEA responds by a strong vasoconstriction to depolarizing agents, to adrenergic stimulation and to products of platelet aggregation, thus emphasizing the need for vasodilators and platelet inhibitors throughout the perioperative period.[10]

INDICATIONS FOR THE USE OF RGEA GRAFT

Indications for the use of RGEA graft include the lack of adequate saphenous vein segments, either because of prior use or because of poor quality of the vein, severe atherosclerosis of the ascending aorta precluding aortic anastomosis,[7,12] and the need for alternative arterial conduits in reoperative CABG for selected patients.[12,13] Lytle and collaborators[14] have enlarged these indications for the use of RGEA grafts to include also young patients with hyperlipidemia because of the poor long-term outcome of vein grafts in this subset of patients.

Advantages to the use of RGEA grafts are a good size match between graft and coronary artery, absence of leg incision, simultaneous harvesting of

RGEA and of internal mammary grafts, possibility of using the vessel as a free graft, avoidance of bilateral internal mammary artery grafting in patients at high risk of sternal infection and, finally, avoidance of side-clamping of a severely diseased ascending aorta.

Disadvantages include the need for a laparotomy incision to harvest the graft and its detrimental effect on postoperative ventilatory mechanics, the risk of epigastric hernia, the technical difficulties of intra-abdominal dissection in obese patients, and the possibility of eventual atherosclerotic disease in coeliac and gastroduodenal arteries. Previous abdominal surgery is only a relative contraindication to the use of the RGEA. Damage to the RGEA graft at an eventual abdominal operation and the resulting acute myocardial ischemia are also of concern for the patient's well-being.

Thus, the use of RGEA grafts is limited by the need for laparotomy, the possibility of coeliac axis atherosclerosis, the limited length of the graft, and by the brittle wall of the artery rendering anastomosis technically difficult. Moreover, patient safety is of concern if further abdominal surgery is required in the future.

Table 1. Angiographic Evaluation of RGEA Grafts

Authors	Year of Report	Follow-up (months)	No. of Grafts Studied	No. of Patent Grafts	
Pym et al[3]	1987	4–24	8	6	(75%)
Lytle et al[14]	1989	1–13	9	9	(100%)
Mills et al[16]	1989	1	29	29	(100%)
Verkkala et al[17]	1989	1	11	9	(81%)
Siclari et al[13]	1990	5	5	5	(100%)
Suma et al[15]	1991	2	46	44	(96%)

CLINICAL RESULTS OF RGEA GRAFTING

Clinical follow-up has not shown any detrimental effects due to the use of the RGEA for coronary grafting, although there is no prospective study and only limited data are yet available. The complication rate is low in all series, and specific complications due to the abdominal part of the operation have been rare events.[15] According to Suma and coworkers,[15] there is no additional risk of early mortality and morbidity with the use of RGEA grafts.

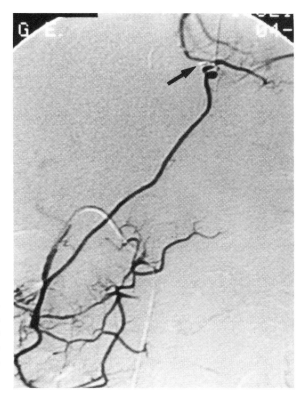

Figure 1. Angiogram of a right gastroepiploic artery graft to the posterior descending coronary artery. (Arrow = coronary anastomosis).

ANGIOGRAPHIC STUDIES

Angiographic studies of RGEA grafts have shown a short-term patency of nearly 90% in small series of patients (Table 1, Figure 1).[14-17] No systematic long-term angiographic evaluation of RGEA grafts has yet been reported.

TECHNICAL CONSIDERATIONS

The median sternal incision is extended down into an upper midline laparotomy incision, after dissection of internal mammary artery pedicles. The RGEA is dissected free from the pylorus to half-way along the greater curvature of the stomach and all arterial and venous side-branches are ligated (Figure 2). The RGEA graft is routed behind, or in front of the stomach and liver, through a window in the diaphragm, to reach the pericardial cavity. The choice of abdominal route is dictated by the length of the graft to obtain the longest graft pedicle with minimal traction. Most often, it is routed behind the stomach, through the lesser sac. The left lobe of the liver is freed from the diaphragm by section of the left triangular ligament, being careful not to damage the spleen during dissection. An incision of 2 to 3 cm in the diaphragm, in front and slightly to the left of the esophageal orifice, is done to access the pericardial cavity at the inferior surface of the heart, near the proximal third of the posterior descending coronary artery. The graft is then

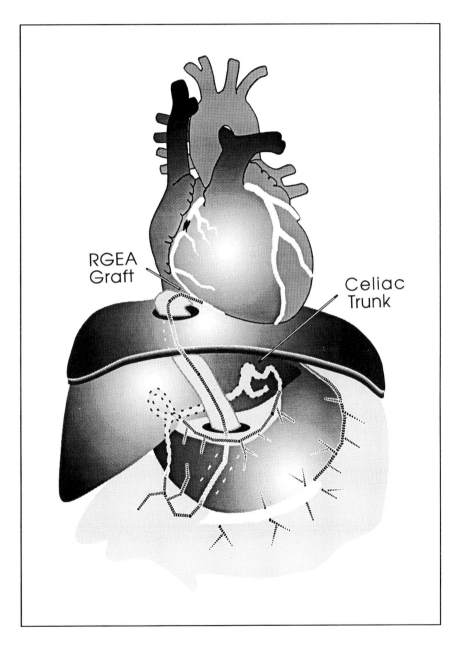

Figure 2. Schematic representation of the surgical technique of right gastroepiploic artery grafting. (RGEA = right gastroepiploic artery).

routed toward the target coronary artery, usually the posterior descending artery. The RGEA to coronary artery anastomosis is constructed with a 8-0 prolene running suture. Topical and intraluminal graft infusion of papaverine has been recommended to relieve spasm due to the dissection, but this must be done with great care to avoid trauma to the graft wall.[16,18]

INITIAL EXPERIENCE AT THE MONTREAL HEART INSTITUTE

Since December 1989, the RGEA has been used as an in situ graft for coronary grafting in 51 patients, 50 men and 1 woman, with a mean age of 50 years. Six of the patients had undergone previous abdominal surgery and two had previously had coronary artery surgery. Saphenous veins were available in all of these patients. There was a triple-vessel coronary disease in 41 patients and a double-vessel disease in 10. Moderate to severe left ventricular dysfunction was present in eight patients.

The same harvesting technique as described above was used in all patients and the retrogastric route was most often chosen. In addition to RGEA grafting, bilateral internal mammary artery grafts were also used in 50 patients (98%) and additional saphenous vein grafts in eight patients. The number of grafted coronary vessels averaged three per patient. The aortic cross-clamp time averaged 77 ± 21 minutes, mean cardiopulmonary bypass time was 113 ± 27 minutes, and overall duration of the operation averaged 278 ± 69 minutes.

There was no operative mortality, and perioperative myocardial infarction occurred in one patient (2%). One patient required a splenectomy because of iatrogenic tear of the spleen during dissection of the RGEA. There was no evidence of phrenic nerve paresis or of diaphragmatic damage following operation. The endotracheal tube was removed the next day following surgery, and oral feeding resumed on the second postoperative day. The average duration of hospital stay was 8 ± 2 days.

Selective RGEA angiography was performed within the first month following surgery in 31 of the patients (62%). The RGEA graft was patent in 28 (90%), two grafts were occluded (6%), and one could not be visualized because of technical difficulties. An angiogram was also obtained one year after surgery in five patients and showed a patent RGEA graft in four of them.

Prolonged gastric drainage, prolonged respiratory support and sternal or abdominal wound complications have not occurred in our experience. No gastric complications were observed and the overall hospital stay was short. Perioperative mortality and morbidity were low, and early graft patency and clinical outcome were satisfactory.

The major limiting factor to the routine use of RGEA remains the lack of data on long-term clinical results and graft patency.[19,20] Therefore, the use of RGEA grafts should probably be restricted for the time being to limited groups of well-selected patients for whom the benefit of using solely arterial conduits for myocardial revascularization is considered essential for a good long-term outcome, or when alternative conduits are not available, until more data on the late patency and efficacy of this graft are available.

THE INFERIOR EPIGASTRIC ARTERY (IEA) GRAFT

ANATOMY, HISTOLOGY AND PHYSIOLOGY

Puig and coauthors[4] introduced the use of the IEA graft in coronary artery bypass grafting in 1988. The IEA originates from the medial aspect of the external iliac artery, approximately 1 cm above the inguinal ligament. It travels superomedially behind the transversalis fascia to the lateral border of the rectus abdominis muscle and enters the rectus sheath midway between the pubis and the umbilicus. It gives off numerous pubic, muscular perforators and cutaneous branches, and it communicates end-to-end with the superior epigastric artery above the umbilicus. This artery averages 3.4 mm in external diameter at its point of origin.[21] The IEA has three anatomic patterns above the arcuate line: a single intramuscular ascending artery in 29% of the cases, two ascending arteries in 57% and three ascending branches in 14%. The anatomy of this artery is usually not symmetrical on both sides.[22]

The IEA is a muscular artery similar to the RGEA, with a media containing smooth muscle cell and vasa vasorum confined to the adventitia, a feature thought to decrease the occurrence of atherosclerosis.[23,24] The media of the internal mammary artery contains more elastic fibers than muscular arteries, which could explain the extremely low incidence of atherosclerosis in the former. The IEA appears to display a moderate tendency for intimal thickening and hyperplasia.[25] Narrowing and gross plaque formation in the proximal 1 to 3 cm of IEA grafts have been reported by Puig and his colleagues[4] and by the group of Barner.[26] However, the precise incidence of atherosclerosis in IEA grafts remains yet unknown.

The useful length of the IEA graft varies from 8 to 13 cm, although grafts up to 20 cm in length have been found.[27] The proximal lumen diameter varies from 2.5 to 3.5 mm and the distal diameter is 1.5 to 2.5 mm.[4,26,28] In Barner's study,[26] the flow through IEA grafts averages 50 ml/min, whereas flows ranging from 80 to 150 ml/min have been obtained after coronary anastomosis and release of the aortic cross-clamp by Puig and his group.[4]

Preoperative evaluation of the IEA by noninvasive testing with duplex scan has been advocated to insure adequacy of the graft before harvesting.[29,30]

Table 2. Angiographic Evaluation of IEA Grafts

Authors	Year of Report	Follow-up (months)	No. of Grafts Studied	No. of Patent Grafts	
Puig et al[4]	1990	1	17	15	(88%)
Buche et al[24]	1992	1	61	59	(97%)
		6	19	17	(89%)

Early bifurcation and small caliber of the vessel can be detected in this way, thus avoiding unnecessary additional incisions. There is a good correlation between the diameter of the IEA at noninvasive duplex scan and that found at surgery.[31] Preoperative angiographic evaluation of the IEA was done routinely in the series of Buche and collaborators,[24] but this appears to be an overly aggressive approach only to obtain information about suitability of the IEA for coronary artery grafting.

CLINICAL INDICATIONS FOR IEA GRAFTS

The IEA graft was initially proposed for patients in whom internal mammary artery or saphenous vein grafts were not available. Excellent early clinical results prompted Puig's group[4] to extend the use of IEA grafts to young patients with hyperlipidemia and to diabetic patients for whom it was desirable to achieve complete myocardial revascularization with arterial grafts only, to avoid vein graft disease.

Advantages of the use of the IEA include the possibility of obtaining two grafts that can be harvested simultaneously with the internal mammary arteries. Contrary to the RGEA, obesity is not a contraindication to its use. The thicker wall of the IEA makes manipulations easier than with the RGEA and decreases the risk of surgical trauma. Disadvantages to its use include the need for abdominal incision and the uncertain quality and length of the graft until it is completely dissected.

CLINICAL RESULTS OF IEA GRAFTING

Early mortality and morbidity in IEA graft series have been low and no ischemic events related to IEA grafts have been reported so far. Abdominal wall hematomas are not uncommon,[26,28] and in the experience of Mills and his group[28] with 74 patients, surgical drainage has been necessary in four cases (5%). Necrosis of the abdominal wall has also been reported in one patient who underwent quadruple bypass with two internal mammary arteries and two IEA grafts.[26] Care must be taken to avoid injury to the ductus deferens during dissection of the origin of the artery.

Early postoperatively, Puig and collaborators[4] obtained a patency rate of 88% among 17 grafts, and the group of Buche[24] found a 97% patency rate in 61 grafts (Table 2). At six months, their patency rate of 19 studied grafts was 89%.

TECHNICAL CONSIDERATIONS

Many surgical approaches and incisions have been proposed to harvest the IEA (Figure 3). Two separate incisions were initially favored by the group of Puig[4] and by Vincent and coauthors,[27] one parallel to the inguinal ligament to explore the IEA and one paramedian infra-umbilical incision to harvest the graft if it is satisfactory. A midline incision has been used to harvest both the right and the left IEA. A paramedian curvilinear incision, starting lateral to the umbilicus and curving towards the inguinal region with lateral or medial

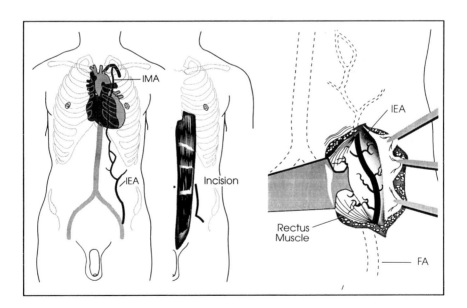

Figure 3. Schematic representation of the surgical anatomy (left), surgical incision (middle) and harvesting (right) of inferior epigastric artery graft. (IMA = internal mammary artery, IEA = inferior epigastric artery, FA = femoral artery).

retracting of the rectus muscle, has been advocated by Milgalter and his group.[30]

The IEA is dissected free from the abdominal wall with a fat pedicle to avoid intimal damage, with the resulting intimal hyperplasia.[23] The free graft is then properly oriented and marked on one side with a sterile ink marker to avoid twisting of the graft. To insure optimal graft size, it is dilated smoothly at low pressure with a papaverine solution. Excision of the IEA with an oval cuff of iliac artery of 4 to 5 mm in diameter has been suggested by Vincent and collaborators[27] to facilitate proximal aortic anastomosis by creating a naturally tapered graft take-off.

Meticulous hemostasis before abdominal wound closure is mandatory to avoid wound hematoma due to systemic heparinization. Delaying wound closure till the end of the procedure has also been recommended.

The IEA has been used to graft all proximal main coronary vessels. Buche and colleagues[24] have used this graft mainly for the proximal right coronary artery. The distal coronary anastomosis is constructed with a 8-0 prolene continuous suture, under optical magnification. Sequential grafts and Y-grafts with the IEA have also been reported.[24,26] Proximal aortic anastomosis of the IEA graft is done in a number of ways, including direct anastomosis to a nondiseased aortic site, indirect suturing of the graft to a saphenous vein patch graft on the aorta, and anastomosis with an oval cuff of arterial wall taken from the external iliac artery at the proximal end of the IEA.[24,25,28]

INITIAL EXPERIENCE AT THE MONTREAL HEART INSTITUTE

Since November 1991, 18 patients have had a coronary artery bypass grafting with the use of IEA grafts, 17 men and 1 woman, with a mean age of 52 years. Two patients had a stenosis of the left main coronary artery and the others had significant triple-vessel disease. Left ventricular ejection fraction averaged 58%. Three of the patients had no saphenous veins suitable for coronary artery grafting. The number of grafts averaged 3 ± 0.5 per patient. A free graft with one IEA was done in each patient. Bilateral internal mammary artery grafts were also performed in 17 of them.

The IEA was harvested before heparin was administered, through a left lower paramedian incision, retracting the rectus abdominis muscle medially, and dissecting the pedicle from the border of the inguinal ligament to the level of the umbilicus. A large pedicle was dissected to include the inferior epigastric veins and adjacent fat. The wound was closed in layers with absorbable synthetic sutures. The IEA graft was marked with a sterile felt marker for proper orientation and dilated with intraluminal papaverine infusion. The distal coronary anastomosis was constructed with a 8–0 prolene

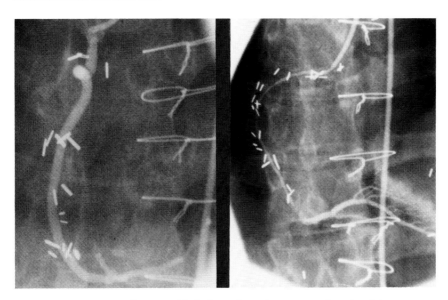

Figure 4. Angiogram of a normal inferior epigastric artery graft to the right coronary artery (left). Angiogram of a small and irregular inferior epigastric artery graft oneweek after surgery (right).

running suture, and the proximal aortic anastomosis with a 7-0 prolene running suture.

The IEA graft was anastomosed to the proximal right coronary artery in nine patients, to a marginal circumflex artery in four and to a diagonal artery in the remaining five. The aortic clamping time averaged 54 ± 15 minutes, mean cardiopulmonary bypass time was 103 ± 37 minutes, and the overall duration of the procedure averaged 262 ± 62 minutes.

One patient (5.6%) died from acute renal failure following surgery. There was no evidence of perioperative myocardial infarction in any patients. One patient developed a constrictive pericarditis one month after operation which required total pericardectomy. Three patients suffered surgical complications related to IEA harvesting, hematoma of the abdominal wall in two and retroperitoneal hematoma with hemoscrotum in one, all of which were treated conservatively.

A postoperative angiographic evaluation of the graft was obtained before discharge from the hospital in 14 of the patients. Eight IEA grafts were patent and six were occluded, for a patency rate of 57%. In addition, one patent IEA graft to the right coronary artery showed diffuse wall irregularities suggesting atherosclerotic changes already present in the artery (Figure 4). Four of the occluded IEA grafts were anastomosed to the right coronary artery. However, postoperative clinical evaluation one month after surgery revealed no evidence of recurring angina in any of the patients.

The low patency rate observed in this early experience may be related to the technical learning curve. Puig and his group[4] found that suturing the IEA to a saphenous vein patch graft for the proximal aortic anastomosis significantly improved the early patency rate. In our series, the aortic anastomosis was always constructed directly on the aortic wall, a technique that can be particularly difficult when the ascending aorta is diseased.

CONCLUSION

It is now technically possible to achieve a complete myocardial revascularization with arterial conduits only, by grafting the two internal mammary arteries, the RGEA and the IEA. The long-term benefit of using an internal mammary artery to the anterior descending coronary artery has been clearly established and results in better patient survival.[32] Bilateral internal mammary grafting has been shown to decrease the incidence of recurrent ischemic events.[33] However, long-term results with the use of RGEA and IEA grafts are not yet available. Based on the current early clinical and angiographic data, these grafts should be recommended only for selective indications at this time. The RGEA graft is useful for young hyperlipidemic or diabetic patients, and for those without good quality saphenous vein grafts, with satisfactory results. For the time being, the IEA graft should be restricted to patients in whom no alternative conduits are available, until the patency rate and late outcome of this graft are more clearly established.

REFERENCES

1. Acar C, Jebara VA, Portoghese M et al. Revival of the radial artery for coronary artery bypass grafting. Ann Thorac Surg 1992; 54:652-60.

2. Edwards WS, Blakely WR, Lewis CE. Technique of coronary bypass with autologous arteries. J Thorac Cardiovasc Surg 1973; 65:272-5.

3. Pym J, Brown PM, Charrette EJP et al. Gastroepiploic-coronary artery anastomosis. A viable alternative bypass graft. J Thorac Cardiovasc Surg 1987; 94:256-9.

4. Puig LB, Ciongolli W, Cividanes GVL et al. Inferior epigastric artery as a free graft for myocardial revascularization. J Thorac Cardiovasc Surg 1990; 99:251-5.

5. Saito T, Suma H, Terada Y et al. Availability of the in situ right gastroepiploic artery for coronary artery bypass. Ann Thorac Surg 1992; 53:266-8.

6. Suma H, Fukumoto H, Takeuchi A. Coronary artery bypass grafting by utilizing in situ right gastroepiploic artery: Basic study and clinical application. Ann Thorac Surg 1987; 44:394-7.

7. Suma H, Takanashi R. Arteriosclerosis of the gastroepiploic and internal thoracic arteries. Ann Thorac Surg 1990; 50:413-6.

8. O'Neil GS, Chester AH, Schyns CJ et al. Vascular reactivity of human internal mammary and gastroepiploic arteries. Ann Thorac Surg 1991; 52:1310-4.

9. O'Neil GS, Chester AH, Allen SP et al. Endothelial function of human gastroepiploic artery. Implications for its use as a bypass graft. J Thorac Cardiovasc Surg 1991; 102:561-5.

10. Dignan RJ, Yeh T, Dyke CM et al. Reactivity of gastroepiploic and internal mammary arteries. Relevance to coronary artery bypass grafting. J Thorac Cardiovasc Surg 1992; 103:116-23.

11. Koike R, Suma H, Kondo K et al. Pharmacological response of internal mammary artery and gastroepiploic artery. Ann Thorac Surg 1990; 50:384-6.

12. Suma H. Coronary artery bypass grafting in patients with calcified ascending aorta: Aortic no-touch technique. Ann Thorac Surg 1989; 48:728-30.

13. Siclari F, Heublein B, Schaps D. Total arterial revascularization of the heart using both mammary arteries and the right gastroepiploic artery. J Card Surg 1990; 5:309-14.

14. Lytle BW, Cosgrove DM, Ratliff NB et al. Coronary artery bypass grafting with the right gastroepiploic artery. J Thorac Cardiovasc Surg 1989; 97:826-31.

15. Suma H, Wanibuchi Y, Furuta S et al. Does use of the gastroepiploic artery graft increase surgical risk? J Thorac Cardiovasc Surg 1991; 101:121-5.

16. Mills NL, Everson CT. Right gastroepiploic artery: A third arterial conduit for coronary artery bypass. Ann Thorac Surg 1989; 47:706-11.

17. Verkkala K, Järvinen A, Keto P et al. Right gastroepiploic artery as a coronary bypass graft. Ann Thorac Surg 1989; 47:716-9.

18. Mills NL, Everson CT. Technical considerations for use of the gastroepiploic artery for coronary artery surgery. J Card Surg 1989; 4:1-9.

19. Tavilla G, van Son JAM, Verhagen ADF et al. Retrograde versus antegrade routing and histology of the right gastroepiploic artery. Ann Thorac Surg 1992; 53:1057-61.

20. Suma H, Takeuchi A, Hirota Y. Myocardial revascularization with combined arterial grafts utilizing the internal mammary and the gastroepiploic arteries. Ann Thorac Surg 1989; 47:712-5.

21. Boyd JB, Taylor GI, Corlett R. The vascular territories of the superior epigastric and the deep inferior epigastric systems. Plast Reconstr Surg 1984; 73:1-14.

22. Moon HK, Taylor GI. The vascular anatomy of rectus abdominis musculocutaneous flaps based on the deep superior epigastric system. Plast Reconstr Surg 1987; 82:815-29.

23. van Son JAM, Smedts F, Vincent JG et al. Comparative anatomic studies of various arterial conduits for myocardial revascularization. J Thorac Cardiovasc Surg 1990; 99:703-7.

24. Buche M, Schoevaerdts JC, Louagie Y et al. Use of the inferior epigastric artery for coronary bypass. J Thorac Cardiovasc Surg 1992; 103:665-70.

25. van Son JAM, Vincent JG, Smedts F et al. Inferior epigastric artery as a free graft for myocardial revascularization (Letter to the Editor). J Thorac Cardiovasc Surg 1991; 101:944-6.

26. Barner HB, Naunheim KS, Fiore AC et al. Use of the inferior epigastric artery as a free graft for myocardial revascularization. Ann Thorac Surg 1991; 52:429-37.

27. Vincent JG, van Son JAM, Skotnicki SH. Inferior epigastric artery as a conduit in myocardial revascularization: The alternative free graft. Ann Thorac Surg 1990; 49:323-5.

28. Mills NL, Everson CT. Technique for use of the inferior epigastric artery as a coronary bypass graft. Ann Thorac Surg 1991; 51:208-14.

29. Milgalter E, Laks H, Elami A et al. Preoperative duplex scan assessment of the inferior epigastric artery as a coronary bypass conduit. Ann Thorac Surg 1991; 52:567-8.

30. Milgalter E, Laks H. A technique to harvest the inferior epigastric arteries for coronary bypass procedures. J Card Surg 1991; 6:306-10.

31. Milgalter E, Pearl JM, Laks H et al. The inferior epigastric arteries as coronary bypass conduits: Size, peroperative duplex scan assessment of suitability, and early clinical experience. J Thorac Cardiovasc Surg 1992; 103:463-5.

32. Loop FD, Lytle BW, Cosgrove DM et al. Influence of the internal mammary graft on the 10-year survival and other cardiac events. N Engl J Med 1986; 314:1-6.

33. Fiore AC, Naunheim KS, Dean P et al. Results of internal thoracic artery grafting over 15 years: Single vs double grafts. Ann Thorac Surg 1990; 49:202-9.

CHAPTER 5

ARE THERE OTHER ALTERNATIVE CONDUITS TO CONSIDER FOR CORONARY ARTERY GRAFTING?

Louis Perrault
L. Conrad Pelletier
Michel Carrier

In exceptional patients the standard and well accepted grafts for coronary artery bypass are not sufficient to meet the needs in regard to the number of grafts to be performed or are simply not available, either because of previous surgical procedures or because they lack the quality required to serve as bypass conduits. This may occur particularly in patients who have already undergone several operations for coronary artery grafting, or when a radical saphenectomy has been performed because of varicose veins. One may then have to consider the use of one of the unconventional alternative conduits. Precise understanding of the risk/benefit ratio of such unusual grafts in myocardial revascularization then becomes a major issue in this decision making.

Obviously, these conduits are contemplated only as a last choice, after all other more dependable grafts, with firmly established clinical value that has stood the test of time, have been exhausted. These include the various conduits already discussed in previous chapters: long and short saphenous veins, internal mammary arteries and the right gastroepiploic artery. Alternative conduits, for which published experience with their use in coronary artery surgery is currently available, are reviewed to determine their clinical usefulness and the role they may currently have in myocardial revascularization (Table 1).

Table 1. *Unconventional Conduits for Coronary Artery Bypass Grafting*

- **Arterial Grafts:**
  - radial artery
  - splenic artery
  - lateral costal artery
  - bovine arterial heterograft
- **Vein Grafts:**
  - lower limb varicose veins
  - upper limb veins
  - human umbilical veins
  - fresh and preserved homologous vein grafts
- **Synthetic Grafts:**
  - dacron grafts
  - polytetrafluoroethylene grafts

ARTERIAL CONDUITS

THE RADIAL ARTERY

The radial artery was first proposed for coronary artery bypass grafting 20 years ago, by Carpentier and collaborators.[1] Several advantages over saphenous vein grafts were stressed by the proponents. The superficial position of the artery made harvesting easy, and a mean length of 22 cm could be obtained. Graft handling and anastomosis were made easier by the wall structure, resistance and elasticity of the radial artery. The smooth endothelial surface, the regular lumen, and its average size of 2 to 2.5 mm which was optimal for coronary grafting, plus the fact that the vessel was physiologically adapted to arterial flow were thought to be features that might offer a suitable solution to the problem of subintimal fibrous hyperplasia that was then often observed in saphenous vein grafts. In addition, in a study of 50 specimens, it was observed that the radial artery was rarely affected by atherosclerotic disease. The authors also stressed that if collateral circulation from the ulnar artery was well developed, as established by preoperative testing, radial artery interruption did not cause hand ischemia.

The initial experience of this group with 40 radial artery grafts in 30 patients indicated a patency rate of 100%, 1 to 10 months following surgery.[1] Narrowing of the graft, attributed to spasm of the artery after its removal, was observed in three patients. In the latter, the radial graft had not been dilated before anastomosing. The authors concluded that to prevent such narrowings, radial artery grafts had to be mechanically dilated after harvesting. Another patient developed a stenosis at the aortic anastomosis attributed to a thick aortic wall. To avoid the difficulty of anastomosing the radial artery directly to a thick-walled ascending aorta, it has been proposed to use it as the distal part of a composite saphenous vein-radial artery graft.[2] With this technique, no evidence of narrowing at the proximal anastomosis of the radial artery was observed on postoperative angiograms.

These early favorable results were soon obscured by other reports on a total of 82 radial artery grafts with a failure rate of 50 to 65% during the first year after operation.[3,4] Curtis and coworkers[3] compared their results with radial artery grafts to those with internal mammary artery and saphenous vein grafts in the same patients.[3] Whereas 82% of internal mammary grafts and 92% of saphenous vein grafts were patent and normal at postoperative angiographic study, only 35% of the 34 radial artery grafts were so. These poor results were not due to unfavorable coronary artery runoff nor to the severity of coronary stenosis,[4] but were attributed to severe and diffuse intimal hyperplasia of the grafts.[3] This is supported by experimental evidence suggesting that fibrous subintimal hyperplasia is a degenerative repair response to ischemic medial necrosis due to the loss of functional vasa vasorum in free arterial grafts.[5] In contrast to the internal mammary artery, which is predominantly an elastic vessel, the radial artery is a thick-walled muscular artery, a characteristic that may predispose to medial ischemia and diffuse spasm, both of which may play a significant role in the early occlusion of the graft.[1,6] From these data, it was therefore concluded that the radial artery should not be considered as a suitable conduit for coronary artery bypass.

Nevertheless, lately there has been a renewed interest in this arterial graft. In a series of 122 radial artery grafts performed in 104 patients undergoing coronary revascularization, Acar and his colleagues[7] found that all grafts were patent within one month of surgery, and that 93.5% of them remained patent after 6 to 13 months. To explain the discrepancy between their excellent results and the inadequate patency rates of previous reports, the authors speculate that the intimal hyperplasia which plagued earlier studies was mainly due to intimal injury during harvesting, causing graft spasm and turbulent flow. There are recent experimental data indicating that in addition to intimal thickening, which can be observed as early as two weeks postoperatively, hypercontractility of free muscular arterial grafts as evidenced by an increase in sensitivity to catecholamines may be the source of problems in those free grafts and result in their occlusion.[8] Although it is not known whether the hyperplastic intima retains any or part of the normal endothelial function, it has been shown that regenerated endothelium of porcine coronary arteries has a decreased responsiveness to endothelium-derived relaxing factors.[9]

If this observation proves to be true also in the human, it might have a significant bearing on the behavior of thick-walled arterial grafts.

Although from a surgical standpoint the radial artery may represent a handy conduit that is easily obtained for coronary artery grafting, and despite the recent more encouraging short-term data, confirmation of these results with further long-term clinical and angiographic studies, and a more definitive understanding of the durability of this graft are needed before the radial artery can be recommended as an acceptable alternative conduit for coronary artery bypass.

THE SPLENIC ARTERY

The splenic artery has been used as an in situ graft to the right coronary artery in a small number of patients, with satisfactory immediate clinical results, and its patency was shown in five out of six grafts studied within one month of surgery.[10,11] The technique of harvesting is more difficult and splenectomy has been necessary.[12] The splenic artery is often tortuous and irregular, and the distance to the coronary arteries is quite long. In addition, a significant incidence of atherosclerotic changes has been found in this artery. In a study of 103 cadavers by Larsen and collaborators,[13] atherosclerotic disease was present in 44 splenic arteries, for an incidence of 43%, compared to 7% in the gastroduodenal artery, and to 86% in coronary arteries. For all these reasons and because of the lack of sufficient clinical experience and knowledge of its late outcome, the splenic artery appears not to be suitable for coronary artery grafting and its use is currently not recommended.

THE LATERAL COSTAL ARTERY

The lateral costal artery is a branch of the internal mammary artery found in approximately 25% of the population. Its use for coronary artery grafting has recently been described in one patient,[14] but there is currently no clinical nor angiographic data to support its use in coronary artery grafting.

BOVINE ARTERIAL HETEROGRAFT

Bovine internal mammary artery grafts are harvested from cows, treated with dialdehyde, and sterilized with ethanol and propylene oxide. These immunologically inert heterografts have been implanted in a small number of patients since 1990. Mitchell and coworkers[15] recently reported their clinical experience with 18 patients. Among a total of 26 bovine arterial grafts implanted, 19 were studied angiographically 3 to 23 months after operation. Only three of the grafts, or 16%, were found to be patent after an average follow-up of 9.5 months, compared to patency rates of 85% for internal mammary artery grafts, and of 75% for saphenous vein grafts, in the same patients. The authors conclude that the intimal surface of the graft is probably thrombogenic, due to the lack of living endothelial cells, and therefore that its poor patency is not surprising. With such dismal results, they do not recommend further use of this bovine arterial heterograft.

VEIN CONDUITS

VARICOSE VEINS OF THE LOWER LIMB

Varicose veins have usually been considered inadequate for coronary artery grafting, because of the risk of aneurysmal dilatation and of rupture of the graft. Vincent and colleagues[16] have reported a limited experience with the use of lower limb varicose veins wrapped in a Dardik net to reshape the vein into a cylindrical tube of more normal configuration and diameter. They contended that the endothelial layer of such veins was still preferable to that of synthetic or biological grafts, and that better patency rates could be expected. Seven patients underwent coronary bypass with the use of this graft with a satisfactory clinical outcome. In four patients studied early postoperatively, all grafts were shown to be patent at angiography. Although the published experience with varicose veins is extremely scanty, it is a common observation that in patients with varicosities of the saphenous vein system, it is often possible to find vein segments with a more normal wall structure that can be used successfully for coronary grafting. In these patients, exploring the short saphenous veins may be worthwhile. However, it must be stressed that when varicose veins are the result of deep thrombophlebitis with postphlebitic syndrome, their harvesting is absolutely contraindicated.

ARM VEINS

The cephalic and basilic veins have been used as conduits for coronary artery grafting after satisfactory early results had been obtained in peripheral vascular procedures.[17,18] However, several disadvantages are associated with their use, including the fragility of the vein wall and the frequent trauma to the vein by previous intravenous injections, the more difficult surgical dissection, and the wound on the forearm that is not cosmetic. Nevertheless, arm veins have been considered by some as the only alternative venous conduit of any value.[19] Early satisfactory clinical results and patency rates were in support of this opinion, even though the quality of the graft lumen was often not optimal.

The available length of the cephalic vein is usually adequate to serve as a graft, as is its internal diameter which varies from 4 to 10 mm. However, in approximately 20% of the patients in whom it was explored surgically, the vein was found unsuitable for coronary grafting.[19] Localized areas of stenosis, irregularity of the graft lumen and aneurysmal dilatations have been described on postoperative angiograms and have been incriminated in the failure of the graft.[20,21] Despite its acceptable early patency rate, ranging from 87 to 90%, the late success rate has been discouragingly low, with only 45 to 50% of the grafts remaining patent without significant stenosis beyond two years.[19-21] There is an almost linear attrition rate of the grafts between one and four years, and the probability of patency at six years is less than 10%.[20] A recent study comparing patients with arm vein grafts to a matched group of patients with saphenous vein grafts found the former to have a significantly lower patency rate and a much greater need for antianginal medication than the latter.[22] After a mean follow-up of 4.5 years, 47% of arm vein grafts remained patent compared to 77% of saphenous vein grafts. The experience with arm vein grafts in coronary artery surgery is similar to that reported for lower limb revascularization. Schulman and Bradley[18] found a cumulative patency rate of 62, 47 and 31% at one, two and five years respectively, among 41 femoro-popliteal bypass grafts with arm veins; in 16 femorotibial bypass grafts, the respective patency rates were 43, 31 and 15%.

Similar to what is observed in the radial artery, the well-developed vasa vasorum system penetrating deeply into the media of cephalic and basilic veins suggests that the outer two-thirds of the vein wall is dependent upon their presence for its nutritional supply.[23] Therefore, degenerative subintimal fibrous hyperplasia may result from hypoxic injury due to dissection and isolation of the vein graft, thus explaining the unfavorable late results. The high incidence of intimal hyperplastic changes and of late occlusion of this graft warrant a word of caution in its use for coronary artery bypass grafting. Arm vein grafts should only be considered as a last choice.

UMBILICAL VEINS

Silver and his group[24] reported their experience with the use of the Dardik biograft, a gluteraldehyde-fixed human umbilical vein, in 11 patients. Umbilical vein grafts of 4 mm in internal diameter were chosen. Thorough irrigation of the graft, with great care to prevent intimal damage, is essential to wash out the gluteraldehyde solution. Whereas gluteraldehyde-treated tissue is nonantigenic, it contains no living cells and becomes merely a skeleton over which recipient cells may grow. The graft is flexible and the circumferential elasticity is excellent, but it lacks linear elasticity, making precise length measurement of the graft critical.

Six of the 12 grafts studied were patent 4 to 16 months following surgery, a patency rate of only 50% after an average of seven months.[24] Although these authors concluded that the umbilical vein was a valid conduit, this opinion has not been generally accepted, hence the lack of further reports on this graft. Because of the unduly high early occlusion rate, the umbilical vein graft cannot be currently considered suitable for coronary artery grafting.

PRESERVED HOMOLOGOUS VEIN GRAFTS

Veins obtained from living human donors have occasionally been used as an alternative to autologous grafts, when the latter were limited or not at all available. There is a very limited experience with the use of fresh vein homografts. Bical and coworkers[25] used fresh vein homografts, kept at 4°C in a saline solution containing penicillin and stored for less than 24 hours, in four patients. No blood-group matching was done in the selection of donors, and patients were not given any immunosuppressive treatment. Angiographic evaluation of the grafts at 8 to 44 months revealed that only two of the seven grafts (29%) had remained open. This is similar to the findings of Ochsner and his group[26] with fresh allogenic vein grafts for revascularization of the lower limb. They reported an occlusion rate as high as 50% within the first year, and the only grafts that had remained patent for more than six months had been obtained from blood-group compatible donors.

Bical's group[25] also implanted 20 cryopreserved homologous vein grafts, stored in glycerol at a temperature of -40°C for up to two months. Whereas six of the seven grafts studied within three months were patent, all three grafts evaluated at one year or beyond were occluded.

There was no correlation between graft failure and donor-recipient histocompatibility, but severe histologic damage to the vein wall was found after only three weeks of cryopreservation. Cold lesions to the graft wall could explain the high occlusion rate. Tice and collaborators[27] implanted cryopreserved homologous veins in 13 patients. Six of eight grafts studied early postoperatively were patent. However, they experienced four sudden deaths during the first two years of follow-up, which may have been related to acute graft closure. These authors concluded that freezing probably decreased immunogenicity in allogenic vein grafts, and therefore that the latter could be used successfully. Their opinion was disputed by Barner[28] who condemned the use of allogenic vein grafts, despite the fact that experimental work from his group indicated a 50% patency rate, 15 to 42 months after graft implantation for limb revascularization.[29] Bical's group[25] also concluded from their clinical experience that freezing caused tissue deterioration of the intima and media and therefore that cryopreserved vein grafts were not adequate for clinical use.

More recently, Laub and associates[30] reported an early patency rate of 41% in 17 cryopreserved vein allografts. Gelbfish and his group[31] found that only 65% of the 31 grafts studied 8 to 12 days postoperatively, and none of the 13 homografts evaluated between 6 and 12 months were normal, with 11 occluded and 2 stenosed grafts at late evaluation. After one year of follow-up, only 35% of the patients remained asymptomatic. These recent data indicate no improvement over previous reports with regard to the patency rate of allografts, and these authors have recommended avoiding their use. Experimentally, it was found that early graft patency was unaffected by treatment to prevent the immunologic response of the graft, either by cryopreservation or by immunosuppression.[32] Therefore, fresh or cryopreserved allogenic vein grafts are not suitable alternative conduits and should not be contemplated for coronary artery surgery.

SYNTHETIC GRAFTS

In 1976, Sauvage and collaborators[33] were the first to report on the use of a synthetic graft in the treatment of coronary artery disease. A small caliber dacron prosthesis was interposed between the aorta and the right coronary artery and remained open up to 16 months. Subsequently, dacron fabric has been replaced by polytetrafluoroethylene (PTFE) in the development of small caliber vascular graft prostheses. Its use for coronary artery bypass grafting was reported for the first time in 1978, in one patient for whom no other conduit was available.[34] The main characteristics of the PTFE graft are its low porosity and easy handling despite the rubbery consistency. For coronary grafting, a prosthesis with an internal diameter of 3 to 6 mm is adequate; its length has to be measured accurately to avoid kinking of the graft, and precise tailoring of the extremities of the prosthesis is required to construct nicely fitting cobra-head anastomoses. Most reports with this synthetic fabric dealt with isolated cases and short-term evaluation: four out of five grafts were found patent between three and six months,[35] one at 18 months[36] and another at 53 months.[37]

Reporting on 16 patients with 27 PTFE grafts, Sapsford and coauthors[38] found 79% of 14 grafts patent within three months, and a 67% patency rate after one year. In Chard's study,[39] 86% of 28 multiple sequential coronary anastomoses were patent at one week, 64% were still patent at one year, 32% after two years, 21% at three years, and only 14% remained open at 45 months. These results were found unacceptable by the authors. Experimental data suggest that treatment with platelet-inhibitor drugs might improve early patency of synthetic grafts,[40] but to this day there are no clinical studies to

Table 2. Early and Late Angiographic Results with the Various Alternative Conduits

Type of Grafts	Authors	Year of Report	Time of Study in Months		No. of Grafts Studied	Success Rate (%)	
			range	mean		≤ 12 months	> 12 months
Arterial grafts							
Radial artery	Carpentier et al[1]	1973	1–10		40	100%	
	Curtis et al[3]	1975	2–12	7.5	34	35%	
	Fisk et al[4]	1976	1–6		48	50%	
	Acar et al[7]	1992	6–13	9	31	93.5%	
Splenic artery	Mueller et al[11]	1973	< 1		6	83%	
Bovine arterial heterograph	Mitchell et al[15]	1993	3–23	10	19		16%
Vein grafts							
Varicose veins	Vincent et al[16]	1985	< 1		4	100%	
Arm veins	Prieto et al[19]	1984	2–9		10	90%	
			15-78	56	8		50%
	Stoney et al[20]	1984	2–108	25	56		44.5%
	Järvinen et al[21]	1984	1–42	17	31		87%
	Wijnberg et al[22]	1990		55	17		47%
Umbilical veins	Silver et al[24]	1982	4–16	7	12	50%	
Homologous veins	Bical et al[25]	1980	< 3		7	86%	
			8-68	29	10		20%
	Tice et al[27]	1976	1–42	17	8		75%
	Laub et al[30]	1992	2–16	7	17	41%	
	Gelbfish et al[31]	1986	< 1		31	65%	
			6-12		13		0%
Synthetic grafts							
	Yokoyama et al[35]	1978	3–6	5	5	80%	
	Sapsford et al[38]	1981	< 3		27	78.5%	
			12-29	21	9		66.5%
	Chard et al[39]	1987	45		28		14%

support this hypothesis in the human. Present data do not support the use of synthetic grafts for myocardial revascularization.

CONCLUSION

Table 2 summarizes the early and late success rates of all alternative conduits for which published clinical experience is currently available. While in a number of studies an acceptable degree of success has been obtained for the very short term (less than 12 months), the results have been almost uniformly distressing and unacceptable after the first year of follow-up. The best long-term results have been obtained with arm veins by several independent groups, with a success rate of approximately 50% between two and six years following operation. Arm veins would therefore appear to be the only alternative grafts that may be considered as a last resort in threatening situations, when no other conduit is available. These are very unusual circumstances, which in our experience are extremely rare. As a matter of fact, among the 5600 patients who underwent coronary artery bypass grafting at the Montreal Heart Institute between 1985 and 1992, alternative conduits had to be resorted to in no more than two or three occasions, when arm veins were used as grafting conduits. On the other hand, it has been exceptional that patients have been denied the benefit of surgical treatment because of the lack of suitable conduits.

A common feature to all of these alternative grafts is the lack of living endothelial lining. The critical role of endothelial cell function in the regional control of blood flow and in the arteriolar vasomotion has been rightly recognized in recent years. The loss of this vasomotor function might play a significant role in the high occlusion rate of these various grafts.[9] The importance of the role of vascular endothelium in vasomotor control also favors the use of grafts with living endothelial cells whose physiological function is well preserved. Further work in this area may eventually lead to the development of new grafts with living and functional neointima obtained from cell cultures that may offer a better long-term outcome. The significance of endothelial function in vasomotor control and as an antithrombogenic factor will be reviewed and discussed in the next chapter.

REFERENCES

1. Carpentier A, Guermonprez JL, Deloche A et al. The aorta to coronary radial artery bypass graft. Ann Thorac Surg 1973; 16:111-21.

2. Picone VA, Leveen HH, Khan R et al. Reversed saphenous vein with proximal attachment of free radial artery segments. A new approach to coronary revascularization. Vasc Surg 1976; 10:8-12.

3. Curtis JJ, Stoney WS, Alford WC Jr et al. Intimal hyperplasia: A cause of radial artery aortocoronary bypass graft failure. Ann Thorac Surg 1975; 20:628-35.

4. Fisk RL, Brooks CH, Callaghan JC et al. Experience with the radial artery graft for coronary artery bypass. Ann Thorac Surg 1976; 21:513-8.

5. Chiu CJ. Why do radial artery grafts for aortocoronary bypass fail? A reappraisal. Ann Thorac Surg 1976; 22:520-3.

6. van Son JAM, Smedts F, Vincent JG et al. Comparative anatomic studies of various arterial conduits for myocardial revascularization. J Thorac Cardiovasc Surg 1990; 99:703-7.

7. Acar C, Jebara VA, Portoghese M et al. Revival of the radial artery for coronary artery bypass grafting. Ann Thorac Surg 1992; 54:652-60.

8. Massa G, Johansson S, Kimblad PO et al. Might free arterial grafts fail due to spasm? Ann Thorac Surg 1991; 51:94-101.

9. Shimokawa H, Aarhus LL, Vanhoutte PM. Porcine coronary arteries with regenerated endothelium have a reduced endothelium-dependent responsiveness to aggregating platelets and serotonin. Circ Res 1987; 61:256-70.

10. Edwards WS, Lewis CE, Blakeley WR et al. Coronary artery bypass with internal mammary and splenic artery grafts. Ann Thorac Surg 1973; 15:35-9.

11. Mueller CF, Lewis CE, Edwards WS. The angiographic appearance of splenic-to-coronary artery anastomosis. Radiology 1973; 106:513-6.

12. Edwards WS, Blakeley WR, Lewis CE. Technique of coronary bypass with autogenous arteries. J Thorac Cardiovasc Surg 1973; 65:272-5.

13. Larsen E, Johansen A, Andersen D. Gastric atherosclerosis in elderly people. Scan J Gastroenterol 1969; 4:387-9.

14. Hartman AR, Mawulawde KI, Dervan JP et al. Myocardial revascularization with the lateral costal artery. Ann Thorac Surg 1990; 49:816-8.

15. Mitchell IM, Essop AR, Scott PJ et al. Bovine internal mammary artery as a conduit for coronary revascularization: Long-term results. Ann Thorac Surg 1993; 55:120-2.

16. Vincent JG, Van Der Meer JJ, Skotnicki SH. L'emploi d'une veine variqueuse pour pontage aortocoronarien. Ann Chir 1985; 39:409-11.

17. Stipa S. The cephalic and basilic veins in peripheral arterial reconstructive surgery. Ann Surg 1972; 175:581-7.

18. Schulman ML, Badhey MR. Late results and angiographic evaluation of arm veins as long bypass grafts. Surgery 1982; 92:1032-41.

19. Prieto I, Basile F, Abdulnour E. Upper extremity vein graft for aortocoronary bypass. Ann Thorac Surg 1984; 37:218-20.

20. Stoney WS, Alford WC Jr, Burrus GR et al. The fate of arm veins used for coronary bypass grafts. J Thorac Cardiovasc Surg 1984; 88:522-6.

21. Järvinen A, Harjula A, Mattila S et al. Experience with arm veins as aorto-coronary bypass grafts. J Cardiovasc Surg 1984; 25:344-7.

22. Wijnberg DS, Boeve WJ, Ebels T et al. Patency of arm vein grafts used in aortocoronary bypass surgery. Eur J Cardiothorac Surg 1990; 4:510-3.

23. Foster ED, Kranc MAT. Alternative conduits for aortocoronary bypass grafting. Circulation 1989; 79(suppl 1):I-34-I-9.

24. Silver GM, Katske GE, Stutzman FL et al. Umbilical vein for aortocoronary bypass. Angiology 1982; 33:450-3.

25. Bical O, Bachet J, Laurian C et al. Aortocoronary bypass with homologous saphenous vein: Long-term results. Ann Thorac Surg 1980; 30:550-7.

26. Ochsner JL, DeCamp PT, Leonard GL. Experience with fresh venous allografts

as an arterial substitute. Ann Surg 1971; 173:933-9.

27. Tice DA, Zerbino VR, Isom OW et al. Coronary artery bypass with freeze-preserved saphenous vein allografts. J Thorac Cardiovasc Surg 1976; 71:378-82.

28. Barner HB. Allogenic saphenous vein for coronary bypass (Letter to the Editor). J Thorac Cardiovasc Surg 1978; 75:902-3.

29. Kraeger RR, Lagos JA, Barner HB. Long-term evaluation of allogenic veins as arterial grafts. Vasc Surg 1976; 10:121-7.

30. Laub GW, Muralidharan S, Clancy R et al. Cryopreserved allograft veins as alternative coronary artery bypass conduits: Early phase results. Ann Thorac Surg 1992; 54:826-31.

31. Gelbfish J, Jacobowitz IJ, Rose DM et al. Cryopreserved homologous saphenous vein: Early and late patency in coronary artery bypass surgical procedures. Ann Thorac Surg 1986; 42:70-3.

32. Deaton DW, Stephen JK, Karp RB et al. Evaluation of cryopreserved allograft venous conduits in dogs. J Thorac Cardiovasc Surg 1992; 103:153-62.

33. Sauvage LR, Schloemer R, Wood SJ et al. Successful interposition synthetic graft between aorta and right coronary artery: Angiographic follow-up to sixteen months. J Thorac Cardiovasc Surg 1976; 72:418-21.

34. Molina JE, Carr M, Yarnoz MD. Coronary bypass with Gore-Tex graft. J Thorac Cardiovasc Surg 1978; 75:769-71.

35. Yokoyama T, Gharavi MA, Lee YC et al. Aorta-coronary artery revascularization with an expanded polytetrafluoroethylene vascular graft. J Thorac Cardiovasc Surg 1978; 76:552-5.

36. Islam MN, Zikria EA, Sullivan ME et al. Aortocoronary Gore-Tex graft: 18-month patency. Ann Thorac Surg 1981; 31:569-73.

37. Murtra M, Mestres CA, Igual A. Long-term patency of polytetrafluoroethylene vascular grafts in coronary artery surgery. Ann Thorac Surg 1985; 39:86-7.

38. Sapsford RN, Oakley GD, Talbot S. Early and late patency of expanded polytetrafluoroethylene vascular grafts in aorta-coronary bypass. J Thorac Cardiovasc Surg 1981; 81:860-4.

39. Chard RB, Johnson DC, Nunn GR et al. Aorta-coronary bypass grafting with polytetrafluoroethylene conduits: Early and late outcome in eight patients. J Thorac Cardiovasc Surg 1987; 94:132-4.

40. Claus PL, Gloviczki P, Hollier LH et al. Patency of polytetraethylene microarterial prostheses improved by ibuprofen. Am J Surg 1982; 144:180-5.

CHAPTER 6

IS THERE A ROLE FOR THE ENDOTHELIUM IN GRAFT PHYSIOLOGY, PATENCY AND ATHEROSCLEROSIS?

Raymond Cartier

The common goal of all interventional therapeutics in the management of coronary artery disease is the improvement of blood supply to the ischemic heart. This is obtained either by reestablishing blood flow in the native circulation using intraluminal devices such as balloon angioplasty, atherectomy catheter and laser-assisted angioplasty or creating new conduits to bypass the flow obstruction in the native vessel with coronary artery bypass grafting. Coronary artery bypass surgery has the unquestionable advantage of reestablishing the blood flow through vascular conduits lined with healthy endothelium.

The endothelial cell lining of these conduits is responsible for their high patency rate even when the grafted vessel has poor runoff. Over the last decade the endothelium has been recognized as a biologically active organ that governs local vasoregulation.[1-4] In normal conditions the vascular tone is regulated through vasoconstrictive and vasodilating influences that are neurogenically released or blood borne derived. The role of the endothelium in the balanced vascular tone would be to provide the normal vessel with "background" vasodilatation for the purpose of preventing vasospasm by circulating vasoconstrictor agonists.[5-7] Besides these vasoactive properties, the endothelium also metabolizes numerous circulating vasoactive substances and releases antithrombotic substances or activate the coagulation cascade.[6,8-10]

VASODILATING AND ANTITHROMBOTIC PROPERTIES OF ENDOTHELIAL CELLS

The healthy vascular endothelium releases plasminogen activator and antithrombin III promoting fibrinolysis. The latter binds to thrombin released by activated platelets and is an important mechanism of thrombin inactivation.[11,12] Circulating thrombin also binds to a specific surface endothelial protein called thrombomodulin which promotes activation of protein C, one of our natural circulating anticoagulant.[13] Anionic charge on the endothelial cell surface related to the presence of glycocalyx complexes is believed to contribute to the antithrombotic aspect of the endothelium. These complexes are made of glycoproteins and glycosaminoglycans with a high content of heparin sulfate and chondroitin sulfate.[14]

Endothelial cells also release prostanoid compounds such as prostacyclin that has vasodilator effect and also decrease platelet aggregation by increasing platelet cAMP level.[15] Besides these compounds, endothelial cells release nonprostanoid substances known as endothelial-derived relaxing factors (EDRFs) and endothelial-derived hyperpolarizing factors (EDHFs).[1,2,16] The acronym EDHF refers to a group of substances that contribute to vessel relaxation by hyperpolarizing the vascular smooth muscle cells. The nature and the mechanism of action of these compounds are not known.

The only identified EDRF is nitric oxide.[17,18] Nitric oxide (NO) is a highly reactive gas with a biological half-life of 6 seconds that is released extraluminally and intraluminally.[19] It is derived from precursor substance L-arginine by oxidation of the guanidino-nitrogen of argine.[20,21] Extraluminally, NO diffuses rapidly through the smooth muscle cell and activates the guanosine cyclase pathway to increase the cyclic guanosine monophosphate (cGMP).[22-24] This increase in cGMP reduces the calcium mobilization from the sarcoplasmic reticulum, reduces the sensitivity to myosin light chain for calcium, and interferes with receptor-operated calcium channels. All these effects decrease the availability of the intracellular calcium and promote smooth muscle relaxation. Intraluminally released EDRF acts in synergism with prostacyclin contributing to vascular relaxation and promoting platelet disaggregation through a cyclic guanosine monophosphate-dependent mechanism.[25-27] There is a constant basal release of EDRF mostly related to the endoluminal shear stress created by blood circulation. Increased blood flow enhances EDRF release whereas a decrease in flow or oxygen tension will have the opposite effect.[28-32]

Numerous substances can promote EDRF release. Acetylcholine (ACh) is referred to as the gold standard means of inducing EDRF released in isolated arteries through muscarinic receptors activation.[33-35] However its physiological role in vivo is probably limited although there is evidence that endothelial cells can synthesize ACH and participate in EDRF release.[36-39]

Vasoactive compounds released by aggregated platelets such as adenosine diphosphate and triphosphate (ADP, ATP), histamine, serotonin, substance P and thrombin have a dual action on the vascular wall.[40-42] In a normal endothelium they stimulate endothelial cells to release EDRF and then contribute to promote vasorelaxation and increase flow, whereas in the presence of a damaged endothelium, they interact primarily with the smooth muscle through specific receptors and promote vascular constriction.[36,43,44] This dual behavior of the vascular wall has clinical relevance. In normal circumstances, the formation of an endoluminal thrombus will trigger an endothelium-dependent vascular relaxation encouraging the washout of the thrombus and restoration of the blood stream. At the opposite, a morphologically or functionally altered endothelium will enhance thrombi formation by a loss of antithrombotic property and an increased propensity for vasospasm.[45] This should remind the surgeon of the importance of preserving the endothelial integrity of vascular conduits during surgery. Moreover, NO has been shown to inhibit smooth muscle cell proliferation in vitro and then can potentially contribute, in the long-term, to prevent or retard the progression of atherosclerosis in coronary artery bypass grafts.[46]

VASOCONTRACTING PROPERTIES OF ENDOTHELIAL CELLS

Besides their relaxant properties, endothelial cells are capable of releasing endothelial-derived contracting factors (EDCF). Thromboxane A2, superoxide anions, prostaglandin endoperoxides and a polypeptide named endothelin are well recognized as endothelial-derived contracting factors.[47,48] Hypoxia and anoxia also trigger the release of an EDCF that is not prevented by inhibitors of cyclooxygenase pathway. These factors can be released by the endothelial cells in specific situations such as cardiogenic shock, uremia or cyclosporin therapy[49-51] and also in normal physiologic conditions.[52-54]

ENDOTHELIUM OF ARTERIAL AND VENOUS CONDUITS FOR CORONARY ARTERY BYPASS GRAFTING

The vasotonic response of vessels varies according to their nature (artery vs vein) and their location (coronary vs peripheral).[55] Successful preservation of the endothelium of vascular conduits depends on "environmental" conditions. Harvesting technique, type of preservation solutions and duration of preservation are all important features that could affect vascular reactivity of the vascular conduit used for coronary bypass. Chronic conditions such as atherosclerosis, hypercholesterolemia and regenerated arterial endothelium have also been associated with impairment of EDRF and prostacyclin production.[56-59] Numerous authors have conducted experiments on endothelial function to characterize the different conduits used in myocardial revascularization. We present a brief review.

SAPHENOUS VEIN AND INTERNAL MAMMARY ARTERY

Reversed saphenous vein graft and internal mammary artery graft continue to be the optimal conduits for complete myocardial revascularization. Patency rate of these conduits varies from 60% at 11 years of follow-up for saphenous vein[60-62] to 90–95% at 10 years for the internal mammary artery.[60,63] Among factors that may explain these differences in patency rate there are the basal and stimulated releases of EDRF and EDCF in these conduits, the technical manipulations during graft preparation and conduit-propensity to develop atherosclerosis.

Human saphenous vein has a lower baseline rate release of NO than internal mammary arteries as shown by Lüscher and his group.[64,65] Quiescent rings of internal mammary artery (IMA) incubated with methylated amino acid Ng-monomethyl L-arginine (LNMMA), an inhibitor of NO formation, increased by 20% their basal tone whereas quiescent rings of saphenous vein were not affected, indicating that NO is spontaneously released by IMA but not by saphenous veins. Stimulated with agonist of the endothelial L-arginine pathway (ACh, histamine), IMA exhibited better relaxation than saphenous vein which was enhanced in the presence of cyclooxygenase pathway blockers indicating that the IMA endothelium-dependent relaxation is then not only related to a higher NO release but also to prostacyclin and possibly EDHF release. Relaxation to ACh is less pronounced in saphenous veins and this is not only related to a lesser NO release capacity of the vein endothelium but also to the endothelial production of thromboxane A2, a powerful vasoconstrictor which counteracts the effect of NO. Similarly, in saphenous veins, histamine mediates an endothelium-dependent constriction through the release of endoperoxide intermediates (prostaglandin H2) and then counteracts the relaxing effect of NO release. In their experiments Lüscher and colleagues[64] also demonstrated that the vascular smooth muscle reactivity was similar in both vessels and then could not be taken into account for the decreased responsiveness of saphenous vein.

The physiological consequences of these observations are numerous. IMA offers better protection against platelet aggression since it releases larger amounts of NO and prostacyclin. Interestingly, the left IMA has been shown to produce in vitro more EDRF than the right IMA[66] and might explain the better long-term patency obtained with the former in some studies.[67] However, any damage to the endothelial cell will increase the risk of vasospasm to circulating catecholamine or platelet-related vasoactive compounds.[68] On the other hand, the L-arginine pathway is not very active in the saphenous vein and is partly inactivated by a concurrent release of thromboxane A2. These effects will enhance thrombus formation and jeopardize graft patency. Although cyclooxygenase inhibitors might not be effective in protecting flow of IMA grafts, they might help saphenous vein grafts in neutralizing the effect of endothelial release of thromboxane A2, thereby enhancing the effectiveness of NO release.[65]

RIGHT GASTROEPIPLOIC ARTERY

The excellent long-term success obtained with IMA grafts led surgeons to explore alternative arterial vascular conduits for coronary bypass. The right gastroepiploic artery (RGEA) has been used with excellent immediate and short-term patency rates for coronary artery bypass graft.[69-74] The "arterial nature" and the morphological similarities to IMA should confer similar endothelial performance to both conduits. Even though numerous clinical experiences show that the RGEA has a diameter comparable to coronary arteries and a pedicle long enough to be used as an in situ graft, there is evidence that this conduit could more likely develop atherosclerosis.[75] Reviewing specimens obtained from 35 patients, Suma and Takanashi found that RGEA has a higher incidence of intimal hyperplasia than IMA (51% vs 23%) even though incidence of overt atherosclerosis was not increased. With regard to endothelial function, RGEA seems to substantially differ from IMA at least by in vitro assessment.

In vitro, isolated segments of RGEA release EDRF in amounts comparable to IMA.[76] However, RGEA demonstrates stronger contraction to depolarizing agent (potassium chloride), to adrenergic stimulation (norepinephrine) and to aggregating platelet products such as serotonin although relaxation to nitroprusside and NO is similar in both vessels.[76,77] The most significant difference between the two vessels is shown in their specific way to behave when exposed to aggregating platelets. Li and coworkers[78] showed that isolated rings of human and porcine RGEA precontracted with norepinephrine and exposed to aggregating platelets exhibited further constriction that was not influenced by the presence of the endothelium. Furthermore, pre-incubation with thromboxane A2 (SQ-30741) and serotoninergic (ketanserin) receptor antagonists as well as inhibitor of NO formation (Ng-nitro-arginine methyl ester) only partly unmasked this contraction. On the other hand, human and porcine IMAs evoked NO-mediated relaxation in these conditions. The authors concluded that activated platelets could induce pronounced contraction of the RGEA and then could contribute to postoperative spasm of RGEA grafts. They advocated the use of antiplatelet drugs and of vasodilators in order to prevent the vasoconstriction effect of thromboxane A2, serotonin and circulating catecholamines on the RGEA graft.[78]

SAPHENOUS VEIN HARVESTING

Numerous factors such as vasospasm, high perfusion pressure, saline storage solutions and harvesting technique have been shown to induce morphological injury to endothelial cells of vein grafts.[79-82] In animals these changes were shown to be reversible over a period of a few months following implantation.[83] However, others have related long-term functional and metabolic changes to the surgical harvesting technique. Angelini and colleagues[84] have shown that saphenous vein subjected to distension with the patient's own arterial blood pressure instead of being manually distended had a better adenosine triphosphate/diphosphate ratio and prostacyclin production preservation indicating a better preservation of smooth muscle and endothelium. In a different study, using bioassay assessment, the same group demonstrated that standard surgical preparation (including adventitial stripping, side branch ligation and uncontrolled manual distension) was associated with a 70% loss of endothelial cell coverage and a 60% decrease in EDRF release compared to freshly isolated vein. Interestingly, storage of freshly isolated veins in blood caused a time-related reduction in maximal EDRF release whereas veins preserved in lactate Ringers solution maintained their ability to release EDRF over three hours of storage. Others have confirmed similar findings with standard surgical preparation.[85] Although the endothelial cells can regenerate, the functional recovery of regenerated vessels is uncertain and chronic increased production of endothelial-dependent constricting substances has been observed in vitro.[86-89] This could explain occasional reports of angina at rest related to spasm of aortocoronary venous grafts, demonstrated angiographically years after the initial surgery.[90-92] Careful surgical dissection and manipulation associated with an adequate storage solution are then essential to preserve morphological and functional integrity of the saphenous vein endothelium.

IMA HARVESTING

Even though dissection of the IMA does not imply as many manipulations as the saphenous vein preparation, endothelial-cell integrity can be jeopardized during certain "routine" surgical maneuvers. Experimentally, controlled dilatation of human internal mammary artery with balloon catheter results in extensive endothelial damage characterized, at the scanning electron microscopy, by desquamation of endothelial cells with areas of complete denudationwith platelet deposits in these areas.[93] Light microscopy also revealed fenestration of the internal elastic lamina with transmigration of smooth muscle cells. These injuries occurred by inflation alone without shearing the catheter or at a very low shear force (20 g) whereas no endothelial damage was reported in animal vessels exposed to shear tension up to 40 g.[94,95] However, the "probing" alone of the canine internal mammary artery was reported to significantly reduce the prostacyclin and EDRF release which was corroborated by significant endothelial damage by scanning electron microscopy.[96] These observations outline the very fragile nature of the human IMA and the importance of limiting all surgical manipulations to a minimum in order to preserve the functional integrity of the graft.

A common practice of surgeons desirous of preventing perioperative IMA spasm is to use topical vasodilators to overcome surgical trauma. In an interesting clinical study, Cooper and coworkers[97] compared the effects of different drugs currently used on IMA-free flow following harvesting. They concluded that sodium nitroprusside was the most efficient topical drug in relieving perioperative IMA spasm. The latter increased IMA flow by 250% over control, whereas nifedipine, glyceryl trinitrate, papaverine and normal saline increased control flow by 161%, 171%, 87% and 25% respectively. Therefore they recommended topical use of sodium nitroprusside during IMA dissection. In a different approach designed to study in vitro the response of IMA to different vasodilators, Jett and colleagues found that nifedipine was the best relaxing drug when IMA was precontracted with depolarizing (potassium chloride) or adrenergic (norepinephrine) agents.[98] In the latter study, nitroprusside was the second most powerful drug whereas nitroglycerin, isoproterenol and adenosine produced little or no relaxation of precontracted IMA.

Despite the excellent results obtained with IMA grafting, instances of inadequate flow during the perioperative period are reported.[99-102] The etiology of these IMA spasms or low flow state is not completely understood. However, inadequate response of endothelial-injured IMA to circulating catecholamine and to platelet-related vasoactive products can be responsible.[36,43,44,78] These studies indicate that in order to prevent graft spasms and optimize blood flow, endoluminal manipulation of an IMA graft should be prohibited and topical vasodilators such as sodium nitroprusside should be used perioperatively. Sublingual nifedipine or intravenous sodium nitroprusside during the first postoperative hours is probably a better choice than intravenous nitroglycerin alone and should be utilized routinely if patient's hemodynamic allows it.

ENDOTHELIAL FUNCTION AND GRAFT ATHEROSCLEROSIS

Patency rate of venous grafts varies from 87 to 93% in the first month and from 74 to 85% 1 year after surgery. Beyond the first year, the mean attrition rate of venous graft is 2.2% per year.[103] Graft occlusion in the first month is related to thrombosis and electron scanning microscopy has revealed endothelial damage in patent grafts of patients who died during this period.[104] Experimental studies have shown that venous grafts were subjected to subendothelial edema, wall inflammatory infiltration and endothelial cell damage during the first weeks after surgery but reendothelialization occurred in all grafts.[105-107] It is plausible to believe that temporary loss of endothelial function could be responsible for the early vein graft dysfunction and occlusion. Intimal fibrous proliferation occurring in the first year after surgery is a recognized cause of graft attrition during this period.[108,109] Intimal thickening and smooth muscle cell proliferation are initiated along during the process of endothelial regeneration.[110] Mechanical stress induced by flow turbulence accelerates the endothelial cell turnover and accounts for the different morphological aspect and increased number of cells normally found with regenerated endothelium.[86,111] Experimental studies have shown that regenerated endothelial cells did not resume normal function.[86,87] Shimokawa and Vanhoutte[86] have reported a decreased endothelial-dependent relaxation to aggregating platelets in porcine coronary arteries four weeks following mechanical denudation. This endothelial dysfunction was mainly related to a lack of responsiveness to serotonin.[86] The loss of the protective role of the endothelium against the effects of aggregating platelets can be one of the mechanisms explaining the graft failure rate encountered during the first postoperative year. Graft dysfunction that occurs beyond the first postoperative year seems to be closely related to vein graft atherosclerosis.[103,112]

Progression of atherosclerosis is a slow process starting generally by nonobstructive fatty streaks that progress to atherosclerotic plaques. This process seems to be accelerated in vein graft of hypercholesterolemic patients.[108] Eventually these plaques rupture exposing subendothelial areas to aggregating platelets with release of vasoactive compounds promoting thrombus formation and local vasospasm as previously described.[113,114] It has been suggested that atherosclerosis even early in its progression is closely associated to endothelial and smooth muscle dysfunction. Endothelium-dependent relaxation is decreased in animals fed with a cholesterol diet for a period of 8 to 16 weeks.[115] These changes in endothelial responsiveness are restored with the reversal of atherosclerotic lesions.[116,117] A possible explanation of this phenomenon comes from the experimental observation that oxidation of low density lipoprotein causes impairment of the EDRF function in pig coronary arteries and rabbit aorta.[118,119] Moreover in vessels affected with severe atherosclerotic changes, the vascular smooth muscle relaxation is significantly altered.[115] All these changes combined together lead to a complete loss of endothelium-dependent relaxation in atherosclerotic arteries[120] and could explain the constant attrition rate observed in aortocoronary venous bypass through the years of follow-up.

Internal mammary arteries are amazingly resistant to atherosclerosis. Sims and coworkers in a necropsic study conducted on 352 unselected individuals, compared the intimal thickening of coronary artery to IMA. While no coronary vessel was free of intimal thickening after three years of age, no significant intimal hyperplasia was seen before the fifth decade in the IMA.[121] This natural protection against atherosclerosis combined with its great ability to release NO and prostacyclin explain the long-term patency of the IMA coronary bypass graft. Furthermore, NO inhibits smooth muscle cell mitogenesis in vitro and differences in its production can explain the high incidence of fibrointimal hyperplasia and of atherosclerotic changes in veins compared to IMA grafts.[46]

CONCLUSION

This brief review outlines the critical role of the endothelium in regard to the outcome of vascular conduits used for coronary revascularization. Long-term patency of IMA, RGEA and saphenous vein graft bypasses is directly bound to the preservation of the specific properties of their endothelium. Careful surgical technique and specific pharmacologic manipulations are imperative to enhance the long-term patency of coronary bypass and then optimize the patient's outcome.

REFERENCES

1. Furchgott RF, Zawadzki JV. The obligatory role of endothelial cells in the relaxation of arterial smooth muscle by acetylcholine. Nature 1980; 288:373-6.

2. Furchgott RF. Role of endothelium in responses of vascular smooth muscle. Circ Res 1983; 53:557-73.

3. Bassenge E, Heusch G. Endothelial and neuro-humoral control of coronary blood flow in health and disease. Physiol Biochem Pharmacol 1990; 116:77-165.

4. Jaffee EA. Cell biology of endothelial cells. Hum Pathol 1987; 18:234-9.

5. Gryglewski RJ, Botting RM, Vane JR. Mediators produced by the endothelial cell. Hypertension 1988; 12:530-48.

6. Bassenge E, Busse R. Endothelial modulation of coronary tone. Progress Cardiovasc Dis 1988; 30:349-80.

7. Fiscus RR. Molecular mechanisms of endothelium-mediated vasodilation. Sem Thromb Hemost 1988; 14(Suppl):12-22.

8. Searle NR, Sahab P. Endothelial vasomotor regulation in health and disease. Can J Anaesth 1992; 39:838-57.

9. Houdijk WPM, de Groot PG, Nievelstein PFEM, Sakariassen KS, Sixma JJ. Subendothelial proteins and platelet adhesion. von Willebrand factor and fibronectin, not thrombospondin are involved in platelet adhesion to extracellular matrix of human vascular endothelial cells. Arteriosclerosis 1986; 6:24-33.

10. Annamalai AE, Stewart GJ, Hansel B et al. Expression of factor V on human umbilical vein endothelial cells is modulated by cell injury. Arteriosclerosis 1986; 6:196-202.

11. Lollar P, Owen WG. Clearance of thrombin from circulation in rabbits by high-affinity binding sites on endothelium. J Clin Invest 1980; 66:1222-30.

12. Bush C, Owen WG. Identification in vitro of an endothelial cell surface cofactor for antithrombin III. J Clin Invest 1982; 69:725-9.

13. Esmon NL, Owen WG, Esmon CT. Isolation of a membrane-bound cofactor for thrombin-catalyzed activation of protein C. J Biol Chem 1982; 257:859-64.

14. Johnson AR, Schulz WW, Herftz A. Glycoprotein synthesis and endothelial cell function. In: Nossel, Vogel (eds). Pathology of the Endothelial Cell. New York: Academic Press, 1982:229-50.

15. Vane JR, Änggård EE, Botting RM. Regulatory functions of the vascular endothelium. N Engl J Med 1990;323:27-36.

16. Chen G, Yamamoto Y, Miwa K, Suzuki H. Hyperpolarization of arterial smooth muscle induced by endothelial humoral substances. Am J Physiol 1991; 260:H1888-H92.

17. Ignarro LJ, Byrns RE, Buga GM, Wood KS. Endothelium-derived relaxing factor from pulmonary artery and vein possesses pharmacologic and chemical properties identical to those of nitric oxide radical. Circ Res 1987; 61:866-79.

18. Moncada S, Palmer RMJ, Higgs EA. The discovery of nitric oxide as the endogenous nitrovasodilator. Hypertension 1988; 12:365-72.

19. Griffith TM, Edwards DH, Lewis MJ, Newby AC, Henderson AH. The nature of endothelium-derived vascular relaxant factor. Nature 1984; 308:645-7.

20. Palmer RMJ, Ferrige AG, Moncada S. Nitric oxide release accounts for the biological activity of endothelium-derived relaxing factor. Nature 1987; 327:524-6.

21. Palmer RMJ, Ashton DS, Moncada S. Vascular endothelial cells synthesize nitric oxide from L-arginine. Nature 1988; 333:664-6.

22. Gruetter CA, Gruetter DY, Lyon JE, Kadowitz PJ, Ignarro J. Relationship between cyclic guanosine 3':5'-monophosphate formation and relaxation of coronary arterial smooth muscle by glyceryl trinitrate, nitroprusside, nitrite and nitric oxide: effects of methylene blue and methemoglobin. J Pharmacol Exp Ther 1981; 219:181-6.

23. Ignarro LJ, Burke TM, Wood KS, Wolin MS, Kadowitz PJ. Association between cyclic GMP accumulation and acetylcholine-elicited relaxation of bovine intrapulmonary artery. J Pharmacol Exp Ther 1983; 228:682-90.

24. Murad F. Cyclic guanosine monophosphate as a mediator of vasodilation. J Clin Invest 1986; 78:1-5.

25. Alheid U, Frölich JC, Förstermann U. Endothelium-derived relaxing factor from cultured human endothelial cells inhibits aggregation of human platelets. Thromb Res 1987; 47:561-71.

26. Furlong B, Henderson AH, Lewis MJ, Smith JA. Endothelium-derived relaxing factor inhibits in vitro platelet aggregation. Br J Pharmac 1987; 90:687-92.

27. Macdonald PS, Read MA, Dusting GJ. Synergistic inhibition of platelet aggregation by endothelium-derived relaxing factor and prostacyclin. Thromb Res 1988; 49:437-49.

28. Bassenge E. Flow-dependent regulation of coronary vasomotor tone. Eur Heart J 1989; 10(Suppl F):22-7.

29. Benyo Z, Kiss G, Szabo C, Csaki C, Kovach AGB. Importance of basal nitric oxide synthesis in regulation of myocardial blood flow. Cardiovasc Res 1991; 25:700-3.

30. Busse R, Trogisch G, Bassenge E. The role of endothelium in the control of vascular tone. Basic Res Cardiol 1985; 80:475-90.

31. Collier J, Vallence P. Endothelium-derived relaxing factor in an endogenous vasodilator in man. Br J Pharmacol 1989; 97:639-41.

32. Drexler H, Zeiher AM, Wollschläger H, Meinertz T, Just H, Bonzel T. Flow-dependent coronary artery dilatation in humans. Circulation 1989; 80:466-74.

33. Angus JA, Campbell GR, Cocks TM, Manderson JA. Vasodilatation by acetylcholine is endothelium-dependent: a study by sonomicrometry in canine femoral artery in vivo. J Physiol 1983; 344:209-22.

34. Komori K, Suzuki H. Heterogeneous distribution of muscarinic receptors in the rabbit saphenous artery. Br J Pharmacol 1987; 92:657-64.

35. Komori K, Suzuki H. Electrical responses of smooth muscle cells during cholinergic vasodilation in the rabbit saphenous artery. Circ Res 1987; 61:586-93.

36. Houston DS, Shepherd JT, Vanhoutte PM. Aggregating human platelets cause direct contraction and endothelium-dependent relaxation in isolated canine coronary arteries. J Clin Invest 1986; 78:539-44.

37. Burnstock G, Warland JJI. P2-purinoceptors of two subtypes in the rabbit mesenteric artery; reactive blue 2 selectively inhibits responses mediated via the P2y- but not the P2x-purinoceptor. Br J Pharmacol 1987; 90:383-91.

38. Burnstock G. Vascular control by purines with emphasis on the coronary system. Eur Heart J 1989; 10(Suppl F):15-21.

39. Vrints C, Herman AG. Role of the endothelium in the regulation of coronary artery tone. Acta Cardiol 1991; 46:399-418.

40. Lüscher TF, Vanhoutte PM. Endothelium-dependent responses to platelets and serotonin in spontaneously hypertensive rats. Hypertension 1986; 8(Suppl II):II-55-II-60.

41. McGoon MD, Vanhoutte PM. Aggregating platelets contract isolated canine pulmonary arteries by releasing 5-Hydroxytryptamine. J Clin Invest 1984; 74:828-33.

42. Burnstock G. The changing face of autonomic neurotransmission. Acta Physiol Scand 1986; 126:67-91.

43. Cohen RA, Shepherd JT, Vanhoutte PM. Inhibitory role of the endothelium in the response of isolated arteries to platelets. Science 1983; 221:273-4.

44. Houston DS, Shepherd JT, Vanhoutte PM. Adenine nucleotides, serotonin, and endothelium-dependent relaxations to platelets. Am J Physiol 1985; 248:H389-H95.

45. Pearson PJ, Schaff HV, Vanhoutte PM. Long-term impairment of endothelium-dependent relaxations to aggregating platelets after reperfusion injury in canine coronary arteries. Circulation 1990; 81:1921-7.

46. Garg UC, Hassid A. Nitric oxide-generating vasodilators and 8-bromo-cyclic guanosine monophosphate inhibit mitogenesis and proliferation of cultured rat vascular smooth muscle cells. J Clin Invest 1989; 83:1774-7.

47. Moncada S, Vane JR. Pharmacology and endogenous roles of prostaglandin endoperoxides, thromboxane A2, and prostacyclin. Pharmacol Rev 1979; 30:293-331.

48. Katusic ZS, Vanhoutte PM. Superoxide anion is an endothelium-derived contracting factor. Am J Physiol 1989; 257:H33-H7.

49. Cernacek P, Stewart DJ. Immunoreactive endothelin in human plasma: marked elevations in patients in cardiogenic shock. Biochem Biophys Res Comm 1989; 161:562-7.

50. Pohl U, Busse R. Endothelium-dependent modulation of vascular tone and platelet function. Eur Heart J 1990; II(Suppl B):35-42.

51. Bunchman TE, Brookshire CA. Cyclosporine-induced synthesis of endothelin by cultured human endothelial cells. J Clin Invest 1991; 88:310-14.

52. Clozel M, Fischli W. Human cultured endothelial cells do secrete endothelin-1. J Cardiovasc Pharmacol 1989; 13(Suppl 5):S229-S31.

53. Gillespie MN, Owasoyo JO, McMurtry IF, O'Brien RF. Sustained coronary vasoconstriction provoked by a peptidergic substance released from endothelial cells in culture. J Pharmacol Exp Ther 1985; 236:339-43.

54. Boulanger C, Lüscher TF. Release of endothelin from the porcine aorta. J Clin Invest 1990; 85:587-90.

55. De Mey JG, Vanhoutte PM. Heterogeneous behavior of the canine arterial and venous wall. Importance of the endothelium. Circ Res 1982; 51:439-47.

56. Werns SW, Walton JA, Hsia HH, Nabel EG, Sanz ML, Pitt B. Evidence of endothelial dysfunction in angiographically normal coronary arteries of patients with coronary artery disease. Circulation 1989; 79:287-91.

57. Shimokawa H, Vanhoutte PM. Hypercholesterolemia causes generalized impairment of endothelium-dependent relaxation to aggregating platelets in porcine arteries. J Am Coll Cardiol 1989; 13:1402-8.

58. Komori K, Shimokawa H, Vanhoutte PM. Hypercholesterolemia impairs endothelium-dependent relaxations to aggregating platelets in porcine iliac arteries. J Vasc Surg 1989; 10:318-25.

59. Shimokawa H, Flavahan NA, Shepherd JT, Vanhoutte PM. Endothelium-dependent inhibition of ergonovine-induced contraction is impaired in porcine coronary arteries with regenerated endothelium. Circulation 1989; 80:643-50.

60. Grondin CM, Campeau L, Lesperance J, Enjalbert M, Bourassa M. Comparison of late changes in internal mammary artery and saphenous vein grafts in two consecutive series of patients 10 years after operation. Circulation 1984; 70(Suppl I):I-208-I-12.

61. Bourassa MG, Fisher LD, Campeau L, Gillespie MJ, McConney M, Lesperance J. Long-term fate of bypass grafts: the Coronary Artery Surgery Study (CASS) and Montreal Heart Institute experiences. Circulation 1985; 72(Suppl V):V-71-V-8

62. Chesebro JH, Fuster V, Elveback LR et al. Effect of dipyridamole and aspirin on late vein-graft patency after coronary bypass operations. N Engl J Med 1984; 310:209-14.

63. Lytle BW, Loop FD, Cosgrove DM et al. Long-term (5-12 years) serial studies of internal mammary artery and saphenous vein coronary bypass grafts. J Thorac Cardiovasc Surg 1985; 89:248-58.

64. Lüscher TF, Diederich D, Siebenmann R et al. Difference between endothelium-dependent relaxation in arterial and in venous coronary bypass grafts. N Engl J Med 1988; 319:462-7.

65. Yang Z, von Segesser L, Bauer E, Stulz P, Turina M, Lüscher TF. Different activation of the endothelial L-arginine and cyclooxygenase pathway in the human internal mammary artery and saphenous vein. Circ Res 1991; 68:52-60.

66. Pearson PJ, Evora PRB, Schaff HV. Bioassay of EDRF from internal mammary arteries: Implications for early and late bypass graft patency. Ann Thorac Surg 1992; 54:1078-84.

67. Huddleston CB, Stoney WS, Alford WC Jr et al. Internal mammary artery grafts: technical factors influencing patency. Ann Thorac Surg 1986; 42:543-59.

68. Sarabu MR, McClung JA, Fass A, Reed GE. Early postoperative spasm in left internal mammary artery bypass grafts. Ann Thorac Surg 1987; 44:199-200.

69. Pym J, Brown PM, Charrette EJP, Parker JO, West RO. Gastroepiploic-coronary anastomosis. A viable alternative bypass graft. J Thorac Cardiovasc Surg 1987; 94:256-9.

70. Lytle BW, Cosgrove DM, Ratliff NB, Loop FD. Coronary artery bypass grafting with the right gastroepiploic artery. J Thorac Cardiovasc Surg 1989; 97:826-31.

71. Suma H, Fukumoto H, Takeuchi A. Coronary artery bypass grafting by utilizing in situ right gastroepiploic artery: Basic study and clinical application. Ann Thorac Surg 1987; 44:394-7.

72. Mills NL, Everson CT. Right gastroepiploic artery: A third arterial conduit for coronary artery bypass. Ann Thorac Surg 1989; 47:706-11.

73. Suma H, Takeuchi A, Hirota Y. Myocardial revascularization with combined arterial grafts utilizing the internal mammary and the gastroepiploic arteries. Ann Thorac Surg 1989; 47:712-5.

74. Verkkala K, Järvinen A, Keto P, Virtanen K, Lehtola A, Pellinen T. Right gastroepiploic artery as a coronary bypass graft. Ann Thorac Surg 1989; 47:716-9.

75. Suma H, Takanashi R. Arteriosclerosis of the gastroepiploic and internal thoracic arteries. Ann Thorac Surg 1990; 50:413-6.

76. Yang Z, Siebenmann R, Studer M, Egloff L, Lüscher TF. Similar endothelium-dependent relaxation, but enhanced contractility, of the right gastroepiploic artery as compared with the internal mammary artery. J Thorac Cardiovasc Surg 1992; 104:459-64.

77. Dignan RJ, Yeh T Jr, Dyke CM et al. Reactivity of gastroepiploic and internal mammary arteries. Relevance to coronary artery bypass grafting. J Thorac Cardiovasc Surg 1992; 103:116-23.

78. Li X-N, Stulz P, Siebenmann RP, Yang Z, Lüscher TF. Different effects of activated platelets in the right gastroepiploic and internal mammary arteries. J Thorac Cardiovasc Surg 1992; 104:1294-302.

79. LoGerfo FW, Quist WC, Crawshaw HM, Haudenschild C. An improved technique for preservation of endothelial morphology in vein grafts. Surgery 1981; 90:1015-24.

80. LoGerfo FW, Quist WC, Cantelmo NL, Haudenschild CC. Integrity of vein grafts as a function of initial intimal and medial preservation. Circulation 1983; 68(Suppl II):II-117-II-24.

81. Stanley JC, Sottiurai V, Fry RE, Fry W. Comparative evaluation of vein graft preparation media: Electron and light microscopic studies. J Surg Res 1975; 18:235-46.

82. Bonshek LI. Prevention of endothelial damage during preparation of saphenous veins for bypass grafting. J Thorac Cardiovasc Surg 1980; 79:911-5.

83. Quist WC, Haudenschild CC, LoGerfo FW. Qualitative microscopy of implanted vein grafts. J Thorac Cardiovasc Surg 1992; 103:671-7.

84. Angelini GD, Breckenridge IM, Williams HM, Newby AC. A surgical preparative technique for coronary bypass grafts of human saphenous vein which preserves medial and endothelial functional integrity. J Thorac Cardiovasc Surg 1987: 94:393-8.

85. Dhein S, Reiss N, Gerwin R et al. Endothelial function and contractility of human vena saphena magna prepared for aortocoronary bypass grafting. Thorac Cardiovasc Surgeon 1991; 39:66-9.

86. Shimokawa H, Aarhus LL, Vanhoutte PM. Porcine coronary arteries with regenerated endothelium have a reduced endothelium-dependent responsiveness to aggregating platelets and serotonin. Circ Res 1987; 61:256-70.

87. Cartier R, Pearson P, Lin PJ, Schaff HV. Time course and extent of recovery of endothelium-dependent contractions and relaxations after direct arterial injury. J Thorac Cardiovasc Surg 1991; 102:371-7.

88. Lin PJ, Pearson PJ, Cartier R, Schaff HV. Superoxide anion mediates the endothelium-dependent contractions to serotonin by regenerated endothelium. J Thorac Surg 1991; 102:378-85.

89. Shimokawa H, Aarhus LL, Vanhoutte PM. Porcine coronary arteries with regenerated endothelium have a reduced endothelium-dependent responsiveness to aggregating platelets and serotonin. Circ Res 1987; 61:256-70.

90. Victor MF, Kimbiris D, Iskandrian AS et al. Spasm of saphenous vein bypass graft: A possible mechanism for occlusion of venous graft. Chest 1981; 80:413-5.

91. Walinsky P. Angiographic documentation of spontaneous spasm of saphenous vein coronary artery bypass graft. Am Heart J 1982; 103:290-2.

92. D'Souza VJ, Velasquez G, Kahl FR et al. Spasm of the aortocoronary venous graft. Radiology 1984; 151:83-4.

93. Barner HB, Fischer VW, Beaudet L. Effects of dilation with a balloon catheter on the endothelium of the internal thoracic artery. J Thorac Cardiovasc Surg 1992; 103:375-80.

94. Gaudiani VA, Buch WS, Chin AK, Ayres LJ, Fogarty TJ. An improved technique for the internal mammary coronary bypass graft procedure. J Cardiac Surg 1988; 3:467-73.

95. Jorgensen RA, Dorbin PB. Balloon embolectomy catheter in small arteries. IV. Correlation of shear forces with histologic artery. Surgery 1983;93:798-808.

96. Johns RA, Peach MJ, Flanagan T, Kron IL. Probing of the canine mammary damages endothelium and impairs vasodilatation resulting from prostacycline and endothelium-derived relaxing factor. J Thorac Cardiovasc Surg 1989; 97:252-8.

97. Cooper GJ, Wilkinson GAL, Angelini GD. Overcoming perioperative spasm of the internal mammary artery: which is the best vasodilator? J Thorac Cardiovasc Surg 1992; 104:465-8.

98. Jett GK, Guyton RA, Hatcher CR, Abel PW. Inhibition of human internal mammary artery contractions. An in vitro study of vasodilators. J Thorac Cardiovasc Surg 1992; 104:977-82.

99. Jones EL, Lattouf OM, Weintraub WS. Catastrophic consequences of internal mammary artery hypoperfusion. J Thorac Cardiovasc Surg 1989; 98:902-7.

100. Barner HB. Blood flow in the internal mammary artery. Am Heart J 1973; 86:570-1.

101. Mills NL, Bringaze WL. Preparation of the internal mammary artery graft: Which is the best method? J Thorac Cardiovasc Surg 1989; 98:73-9.

102. Sarabu MR, McClung JA, Fass A, Reed GE. Early post-operative spasm in left internal mammary artery bypass grafts. Ann Thorac Surg 1987; 44:199-200.

103. Bourassa MG, Campeau L, Lesperance J, Grondin CM. Changes in grafts and coronary arteries after saphenous vein aortocoronary bypass surgery: Results at repeat angiography. Circulation 1982; 65(Suppl II):II-90-II-7.

104. Kern WH, Dermer GB, Lindesmith GG. The intimal proliferation in aortic-coronary saphenous vein grafts. Lights and electron microscopic studies. Am Heart J 1972; 84:771-7.

105. Brody WR, Kosek JC, Angell WW. Changes in vein grafts following aortocoronary bypass induced by pressure and ischemia. J Thorac Cardiovasc Surg 1972; 64:847-54.

106. Jones M, Conkle DM, Ferrans VJ et al. Lesions observed in arterial autogenous vein grafts. Light and electron microscopic evaluation. Circulation 1973; 48(Suppl III): III-198-III-210.

107. Spray TL, Roberts WC. Status of the grafts and the native coronary arteries proximal and distal to coronary anastomotic sites of aortocoronary bypass grafts. Circulation 1977; 55:741-9.

108. Lie JT, Lawrie GM, Morris GC Jr. Aortocoronary bypass saphenous vein graft atherosclerosis: anatomic study of 99 vein grafts from normal and hyperlipoproteinemic patients up to 75 months postoperatively. Am J Cardiol 1977; 40:906-14.

109. Bulkley BH, Hutchins GM. Accelerated "atherosclerosis": a morphologic study of 97 saphenous vein coronary artery bypass grafts. Circulation 1977; 55:163-9.

110. Schwartz SM, Gajdusek CM, Selden SC. Vascular wall growth control: the role of the endothelium. Arteriosclerosis 1981; 1:107-61.

111. Spagnoli LG, Pietra GG, Villaschi S, Johns LW. Morphometric analysis of gap junctions in regenerating arterial endothelium. Lab Invest 1982; 46:139-48.

112. Campeau L, Lesperance J, Corbara F et al. Aortocoronary saphenous vein bypass graft changes 5 to 7 years after surgery. Circulation 1978; 58(Suppl I):I-170-I-5.

113. Stein B, Fuster V, Israel DH et al. Platelet inhibitor agents in cardiovascular disease: an update. J Am Coll Cardiol 1989; 14:813-36.

114. Ross R. The pathogenesis of arteriosclerosis. N Engl J Med 1986; 314:488-500.

115. Verbeuren TJ, Jordaens FH, Zonnekeyn LL et al. Effect of hypercholesterolemia on vascular reactivity in the rabbit: I. Endothelium-dependent and endothelium-independent contractions and relaxations in isolated arteries of control and hypercholesterolemic rabbits. Circ Res 1986; 58:552-64.

116. Heistad DD, Mark AL, Marcus ML, Piegors DJ, Armstrong ML. Dietary treatment of atherosclerosis abolishes hyperresponsiveness to serotonin: implications for vasospasm. Circ Res 1987; 61:346-51.

117. Bossaller C, Habib GB, Yamamoto H et al. Impaired muscarinic endothelium-dependent relaxation and cyclic guanosine 5-monophosphate formation in atherosclerotic human coronary artery and rabbit aorta. J Clin Invest 1987; 79:170-4.

118. Simon BC, Cunningham LD, Cohen RA. Oxidized low density lipoproteins cause contraction and inhibit endothelium-dependent relaxation in the pig coronary artery. J Clin Invest 1990; 86:75-9.

119. Jacobs M, Plane F, Bruckdorfer KR. Native and oxidized low-density lipoproteins have different inhibitory effects on endothelium-derived relaxing factor in the rabbit aorta. Br J Pharmacol 1990; 100:21-6.

120. Verbeuren TJ, Jordaens FH, Van Hove CE, Van Hoydinck AE, Herman AG. Release and vascular activity of endothelium-derived relaxing factor in atherosclerotic rabbit aorta. Eur J Pharmacol 1990; 191:173-84.

121. Sims FH. A comparison of coronary and internal mammary arteries and implications of the results in the etiology of arteriosclerosis. Am Heart J 1983; 105:560-6.

CHAPTER 7

SUMMARY

Michel Carrier
L. Conrad Pelletier

Coronary artery bypass grafting has come a long way since the early days of 1967. The indications and choice of patients are now well established. It has been firmly demonstrated that the long-term outcome is directly related to the degree of sustained success obtained with the various conduits, hence the importance of appropriate selection of graft material at the time of operation.

All data indicate without any doubt that the internal mammary artery is currently the graft of choice for coronary artery bypass. While the short-term evaluation shows results that are similar to those obtained with saphenous vein grafts, the 10-year clinical and angiographic results have been so much better with the former that it has stimulated interest to search for other arterial conduits that might be used as adjuvants to double mammary artery grafts in order to achieve complete myocardial revascularization with arterial grafts only. This may be particularly relevant for younger patients with a potential for prolonged survival and for those who are particularly susceptible to very aggressive vein graft disease, such as hyperlipidemic or diabetic patients. In this regard, sequential anastomoses with the internal mammary arteries or their use as free grafts have widened the possibilities of achieving a more complete revascularization. The right gastroepiploic artery has offered another interesting possibility in recent years, and may particularly be useful to revascularize the inferior and diaphragmatic territories which can barely be reached with mammary artery grafts.

Saphenous vein grafts will no doubt continue to hold a major place in coronary artery bypass grafting. They currently serve to construct about half of the coronary grafts in our experience, and they will likely maintain this level of use in coming years. However, they now are mainly used to revascularize territories of lesser importance, or as a second choice when mammary arteries are unsuitable or unavailable. In addition to the long and short saphenous veins, arm veins may also be helpful as a last choice when all other conduits have been exhausted, despite their suboptimal long-term results. Among the various alternative conduits, arm veins are the only one that can be proposed at this time with some degree of success, all other arterial, venous or synthetic grafts being unsuitable for coronary artery bypass grafting.

Our better understanding of the functional role of the vascular endothelial cell, which remained unsuspected until a few years ago, has already modified our attitude toward grafts and coronary arteries in a number of ways. More aware of the need to preserve an intact intima, we now avoid manipulations and pressure flushing of the grafts and do not probe or dilate internal mammary artery grafts or coronary arteries, as we used to. The loss of endothelial cell function may also be partly responsible for the dismal results with most conduits used as free grafts, except for the internal mammary artery and saphenous vein, as well as with synthetic grafts. Coming years may bring along new grafts, with living and functional endothelial lining whose long-term outcome may be improve.

Better myocardial protection and continued progress in coronary angioplasty and atherectomy will contribute to further changes in the profile of the population undergoing surgical treatment. Older and more challenging patients because of more severe coronary artery disease and left ventricular dysfunction will come at surgery. On the other hand, a more extensive use of arterial conduits will contribute to stop the progression or even decrease the incidence of reoperations for coronary artery grafting in the future.

The main issue that will have to be faced concerns the socio-economic aspect of the surgical treatment of coronary artery disease. After the questioning of the scientific value of the operation in the 1970's, it will now be evaluated in terms of its sustained social and economical value and of its cost/benefit ratio. This will be the challenge of the end of this century, and surely the choice of the best possible conduit for coronary artery grafting will have a profound influence on the late outcome of the patients and on the assessment of its role in the treatment of coronary artery disease.

INDEX

Items in italics indicate figures (f) or tables (t).